Eat Smart Beat Migraine

Eat Smart
Beat Migraine

Michele Sharp

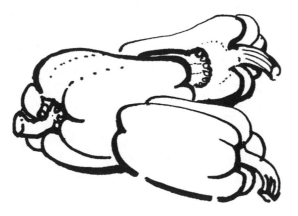

GRUB STREET · LONDON

Published by Grub Street, The Basement,
10 Chivalry Road, London SW11 1HT

Copyright this edition © Grub Street 2002
Text copyright © Michele Sharp 2001
First published by Key Porter Books, Canada
as *The Migraine Cookbook*

British Library Cataloguing in Publication Data
Sharpe, Michele
    Eat smart beat Migraine
    1. Migraine – Diet therapy – Recipes
    I. Title
    641.5'631

ISBN 1 904010 06 7

Typesetting by Pearl Graphics, Hemel Hempstead
Printed and bound in Great Britain by
Biddles Ltd, Guildford and King's Lynn

Contents

1. GENERAL
INTRODUCTION

Acknowledgements	vi
Foreword	vii
More Than Just a Headache	viii
Diagnosis and Management of Migraine	xiii
Managing Dietary Triggers	xix
How to Use This Cookbook	xxv

2. RECIPES

Appetisers and Snacks	1
Soups and Salads	10
Meatless Main Courses	27
Meat and Poultry	35
Fish and Seafood	52
Vegetables and Side Dishes	69
Quick Breads, Desserts and Baked Goods	81
Beverages	113
Basic Stocks and Sauces	120
Resources Directory	126
Bibliography	130
Index	131

ACKNOWLEDGEMENTS

The inspiration for this book must go first to our Fredericton, New Brunswick chapter. They were a wonderful source for many of the delicious recipes. I would also like to individually thank those loyal members, volunteers and supporters across the country who provided support in bringing the various elements of this book together: Joanne Brown; Heather-Ann Brown; Erik Buchanan; Bonnie Buxton; Elaine Comish; Maria Conforto; Pamela Douglas; Laura Eagle-LaDuke; Sylvia Fowles; Edith Freeman; Alice Gauvin; Patti Hanson; Laura Hennick; John Holland; Maura Keenan; Sally Ann Kerman; Lois Lavers; Sara Lawson; Emily Levitt; Meg Lloyd-Jones; Connie Luyt; Arlene Mahood; Elizabeth McKim; Ruth Miln; Victoria Mountain; Bob Olsen; Olga Peacock; Dr. Allan Purdy; Jenny Reid; Dr. Gordon Robinson; Mary-Ann Roebellen; Andrea Rolston; Bill Ross; Nelly Sabbagh; Malcolm Sharp; Nelda Sharp; Dr. Ashfaq Shuaib; Donna-Lynn Turner; G. Joy Underwood; Grace Wood; and Dave Wright. I'd also like to recognise our dedicated volunteer Board of Directors: Georgina Kossivas, Dr. Marek Gawel, Karen Ormerod, Barbara Nawrocki, Dr. Rose Giammario, Dr. Gary Shapero and Debbie Drewett.

Special thanks should also go to Susan Folkins, my editor, for all her patience and advice. Thanks also to Anna Porter, Clare McKeon, Irene Worthington, Dr. Marek Gawel, Valerie South, Liba Berry and Cathy Fraccaro. All of your comments, suggestions and keen support were greatly appreciated.

I'd also like to recognise Astra Zeneca for their commitment to The Migraine Association of Canada and their assistance in making aspects of this project possible.

Many Toronto chefs also generously contributed recipes to our first cookbook, *Fabulous Cooking Ideas*. Some of their recipes are reprinted here. Thanks also to the chefs at North 44 for sharing their delicious recipe for Steamed Basmati Rice. I would also like to thank the authors of *HeartHealthy Cooking*, *Fare for Friends* and *Good Friends Cookbook* for granting us permission to reprint a few of their recipes.

Finally, I would like to thank our invaluable volunteers who provided us with their time, energy and support. We would not be able to continue to provide much needed information, education and services without you!

Foreword

Migraine is one of the most undertreated, misunderstood and misdiagnosed disorders of the last century. And yet it is a serious medical disorder that significantly affects millions of people in the UK. In fact, prevalence studies indicate that 15 percent of the UK population suffer from migraine – somewhere in the region of 9 million sufferers. Also over 10 percent of school age children suffer from migraine. As Rosemary Dudley, the founder of The Migraine Association of Canada, stated "Perhaps no other condition so disrupts the lives of its victims and yet evokes so little sympathy and compassion for the afflicted."

Migraine has a significant impact on an individual's personal and professional life. It can lead to lost work days, hindered job performance, restricted activities and disrupted relationships. Statistics indicate that 90,000 people are absent from work or education every day because of migraine. The cost to the UK economy, in terms of working days lost or people working less effectively during an attack is estimated at around £1 billion annually.

While there is no known cure for migraine, understanding your triggers can help you take charge of your attacks. For those of you who find that certain foods can be a trigger, *Eat Smart Beat Migraine* will help to educate and empower you. It has been designed to make you think more about your lifestyle so that you can recognise patterns that lead up to an attack. Through identifying and eliminating or avoiding your triggers, I hope you will be able to provide yourself with a measure of relief against the terrible pain of migraine.

More Than Just a Headache

Almost everyone has a headache now and then. The most common form of headache is tension type headache. Unlike migraine and other headache disorders, tension type headache is mild to moderate and is usually alleviated with rest and relaxation or over-the-counter pain relievers. Migraine, however, is a neurological disorder that involves a complex relationship between the blood supply to the brain and its nerve network.

Migraine occurs most often among people aged 20 to 50. The most common symptom associated with migraine is severe head pain made worse by routine activities, such as climbing stairs or bending over. The pain, often described by sufferers as 'throbbing,' is commonly felt on one side of the head, although it can switch sides during an attack or from one attack to the next. Many migraine sufferers feel nauseous and some vomit during an attack. Typically, sufferers are extremely sensitive to light, sound and odours, making ordinary events unbearable.

For the majority of migraine sufferers, or migraineurs, an untreated or unsuccessfully treated attack lasts 24 hours, although attacks can vary from two hours to several days. An average sufferer may have as many as 20 attacks every year; however, as many as 9 percent of sufferers experience 52 or more. During an attack and often leading up to and following an attack, migraineurs can become disabled, that is, it is necessary for them to completely or partially restrict their activities.

Migraine is more than a just a headache. In addition to waves of nausea and sensitivity to light, sound and odour, about one-fifth of migraine sufferers experience an 'aura,' a visual or sensory disturbance that acts as a warning sign to the oncoming headache. Other symptoms, often in the period of time leading up to the headache, include: irritability, depression, elation, excessive yawning, difficulty concentrating, dizziness, trouble with words, hyperactivity and food cravings (for more about the symptoms of migraine, see p. xiv).

Why People Get Migraines

Experts have yet to pinpoint the exact cause of migraine, yet they do know it tends to run in families. In fact, over 50 percent of migraine sufferers have a close relative who experiences similar headaches, which indicates that migraine may be inherited. With the discovery of the gene responsible for familial hemiplegic migraine (a very rare form of the disorder), experts believe that with further research they may be able to generalise this information to the broader disorder. In the meantime, leading health experts describe individuals with migraine as wired differently, with a predisposition towards episodic migraine attacks. What triggers individual attacks varies between people and from one attack to the next.

What Happens in the Head

A complete understanding of the complex chain of physical events that precipitate a migraine attack is not fully understood. However, research in the past few decades has led to a better understanding of what happens in the head during a migraine attack. Researchers now know that certain chemicals in the brain – substance P, neurokinin A, and calcitonin gene-related peptide (CGRP), among others – are released and land on blood vessels. These chemicals cause the blood vessels to expand and send signals via the nerves to the brain, where the signals are processed to determine that the sensation is a painful one.

Types of Migraine

The two most common types of migraine are migraine without aura and migraine with aura. There are also several subtypes (atypical migraines) that are quite rare. They present themselves differently from the more common types, but researchers believe the triggers are the same.

Migraine without aura (previously called 'common migraine')

Most migraineurs experience migraine without aura, usually described as throbbing head pain made worse by routine activities, such as climbing stairs or bending over; pain on one side of the head (although it can be on both sides or switch sides during an attack or from one attack to the next); nausea and/or vomiting; or extreme sensitivity to light, sound or smell. People afflicted with migraine frequently describe the pain as 'hammering' or 'pulsating.'

Migraine with aura (previously called 'classic migraine')

As many as 20 percent of migraine sufferers experience an aura before their migraine attack. As explained above, an aura is a visual or sensory disturbance that acts as a warning sign of the oncoming headache. Typical aura symptoms include: flashes of light, blurred vision, or blind spots spreading across the visual field. Some sufferers may feel tingling or numbness in the face, arms or hands. The symptoms usually fade within one hour as they give way to severe head pain. In some cases, however, a headache never follows. These migraine sufferers have migraine aura without headache.

Atypical migraine

There are also uncommon types of migraine such as familial hemiplegic migraine, basilar migraine and ophthalmoplegic migraine.

Familial hemiplegic migraine is the only type of migraine to have had a specific gene identified. This very rare atypical migraine is believed to result from a prolonged profound aura involving the brain. Symptoms often can mimic a stroke or tumor and range from a slight tingling or numbness on one side of the face or body to partial short-term paralysis. The headache is usually one-sided but the after-effects of the aura can last for days. Rarely is it permanent.

Basilar migraine, also known as 'basilar artery migraine,' 'Bickerstaff's migraine' and 'syncopal migraine' is associated with several distinct aura symptoms. They include:

- Visual symptoms such as double vision
- Slurred speech
- Dizziness and/or vertigo
- Ringing in the ears
- Decreased hearing
- Numbness and tingling in limbs on both sides or severe weakness/paralysis of limbs on both sides
- Decreased level of awareness of surroundings

Ophthalmoplegic migraine is a very rare type of migraine. It involves repeated headaches with a paralysis of one or more cranial nerves that control pupil dilation and eye movement. People often experience double vision, and the symptoms may be mistaken for an aneurysm (a ballooning of the blood vessels in the head that can rupture and cause bleeding).

Other types of headache
Medication-induced headaches/rebound headaches
Medication-induced headaches or rebound headaches have become increasingly common. Migraine sufferers are often susceptible to developing these conditions. Scientists believe that when the level of analgesics (pain relievers) begins to lower in the body, the individual experiences a withdrawal reaction in the form of a headache. Increasing the level of analgesics relieves the headache, not because of the painkilling effect, but because it temporarily interrupts withdrawal. This condition can also occur with ergotamines. Only the complete elimination of analgesics or ergotamines in the system will end this vicious cycle. Discuss the options with your doctor.

Cluster headaches
Cluster headaches, another form of headache, should not be confused with migraine attacks. Unlike migraine, which occurs in nearly 15 percent of the UK population, cluster headache occurs in less than 1 percent of the population. Eighty-five percent of all cluster headache sufferers are men.

   The symptoms of cluster headache are distinctly different from those of migraine. Attacks of cluster headache are grouped in a series of short, intensely severe bursts of pain, usually lasting 30 to 45 minutes and rarely lasting longer than four hours. Often occurring at night, the pain is sharp, piercing and debilitating. If you think you might be suffering from cluster headaches, consult your doctor and get a proper diagnosis. Cluster and migraine are distinct disorders with different symptoms and treatments.

Migraine in Women
Before puberty, the prevalence of migraine in both sexes is about equal. However, at the onset of puberty, the incidence of migraines in females increases dramatically. In adults, migraine is three times more prevalent in women than in men. It is believed that this is due to hormonal changes associated with the reproductive cycle.

For women whose migraines start at puberty, their migraines often show a lifelong connection to their menstrual cycle. Migraine attacks are linked to the menstrual cycle in about 60 percent of affected women (menstrually related migraine), and exclusive to the menstrual cycle in roughly 14 percent of affected women (true menstrual migraine). Both forms of menstrual migraine occur during or just after oestrogen levels fall. Since oestrogen levels fall after ovulation and before menstruation, this could account for headaches at these times. Depending on the woman's circumstances, doctors may prescribe hormone replacement therapy (HRT), which helps to stabilise oestrogen levels during these critical times. In addition, some doctors prescribe non-steroidal anti-inflammatory drugs (NSAIDs), such as ibuprofen or naproxen, in the prevention of menstrual migraine.

For many women, their episodes of attacks improve with pregnancy or menopause. However, for some women migraine may appear for the first time during pregnancy. Often migraine will improve during the second and third trimesters, but throughout the pregnancy, and especially during the first trimester, medication must be approached cautiously and should be taken only on the advice of a doctor.

Oral contraceptives, which contain oestrogen and progesterone, can induce, change or alleviate migraine. Their use can trigger the first migraine attack (most often in women with a family history of migraine) or exacerbate existing migraine, especially on those days when the woman is off the oral contraceptive.

During the early menopausal stage, tremendous fluctuations in oestrogen can worsen migraine. Hormone replacement with oestrogen, alone or in combination with progesterone, can either exacerbate migraine or relieve it. Cyclical hormone replacement therapy may trigger migraine in the days off the supplement, so continuous low doses of oestrogen and progesterone are sometimes preferable. According to a recent North American study, 62 percent of women experience fewer migraine headaches and a marked improvement after menopause; 28 percent felt no difference and 10 percent felt their migraines were worse.

Migraine in Children

If you're a parent, guardian or adult caring for a child with migraine, there may be some comfort in knowing that you're not alone. Approximately 10 percent of schoolage children suffer from migraine. While as many as one-third of children will outgrow migraine, many will go on to have migraine in adolescence. After age 12, the incidence of migraine increases in girls due to the role of hormones. By age 14, the rate for girls is approximately 15 percent, while the rate for boys hovers at 6 percent. Approximately 25 percent of adults with migraine report that their symptoms started before age 10.

Migraine in children is unique for several reasons. While identifying migraine in adults can be a challenge, diagnosing it in children is even more difficult. Children communicate their symptoms differently than adults. It's unlikely, for example, that you'll hear a child say, "I've been having a throbbing pain in my left temple accompanied by nausea two times a month." Instead, parents might notice that an otherwise playful child suddenly becomes introverted, irritable or covers his or her eyes.

Naturally, migraine affects children in different ways than adults. Children may miss school, stop participating in social activities, decline invitations to parties and, in some cases, may develop coping and communication problems. Adults caring for children with migraine can play a vital role in early detection, appropriate care, preventive measures and the development of a support network – all of which contribute to a positive attitude towards the disorder and enhance the sufferer's overall participation in life.

Sorting out the symptoms in children can be very difficult. As with adults, the most common form of migraine in children is migraine without aura, characterized by one or two-sided often frontal (across the forehead) moderate to severe head pain; sensitivity to light, sound and smells; and nausea or vomiting. Headaches in children are usually of shorter duration than those in adults. Your child's migraine may last for only one hour, and may be relieved after a long nap. In some cases, migraine can last for as long as two days.

The second most common form, migraine with aura, is characterised by visual or sensory disturbances. Blind spots, difficulty focusing and displays of flashing lights can be especially distressing for children. Other symptoms include numbness or tingling in the arms and hands or around the mouth. Some children will have the aura without the headache, with the possibility of developing the headache later in life.

Additional symptoms, possibly indicative of other types of migraine, such as double vision, eye pain, slurred speech, confusion, and weakness or paralysis, should be discussed with your doctor. Very young children may experience abdominal pain, intense vomiting, loss of balance or the feeling that everything around them is going very fast or very slow, or is unusually big or small. These symptoms may be the first expression of migraine, and can frighten or confuse both the child and adult.

Getting an accurate diagnosis and ruling out other causes is the first step in managing migraine (see p. xvi). Many symptoms will disappear as the child matures and grows out of them, or as the more common features of migraine become more prominent. A visit to the doctor to review the child's history and symptoms will establish whether the child has migraine.

The next step is identifying triggers. No two children have exactly the same triggers, although there are a number of common ones. Susceptibility to triggers will change from time to time, depending on the child's overall emotional and physical well-being. For some children, diet is a key trigger; for others, stress, missed sleep or skipped meals, changes in weather, or changes to routine can bring on migraine. Reducing exposure to triggers is a key strategy for reducing the frequency of migraine.

During migraine attacks, children may find comfort in retreating to a darkened quiet room. Cold packs, fluids in moderation and a short nap may stave off an attack. When non-drug strategies are not successful, medication is an option when used as directed. In pediatric doses, over-the-counter medications such as ibuprofen (for older children or adolescents) or acetaminophen can help alleviate an attack. Acetylsalicylic acid (ASA) should not be used in children 12 years and under because of its association with Reye's syndrome (an often fatal disease of the brain that usually occurs in children following an acute viral infection).

Combination pain relievers containing codeine or migraine-specific medications (such as sumatriptan, zolmitriptan, naratriptan, rizatriptan or eletriptan) may be used in older children and adolescents when all other measures fail. Pain relievers should not be taken more than two days a week, in order to prevent rebound headaches (see p. x).

For chronic attacks or severe pain, hospital treatment and/or preventive medications may be recommended.

In all cases, medication should be taken only at the advice of the child's physician. Some medications on the market have been tested only on adults and may not be suitable to children. Don't share your own or any one else's medication with your child.

It is important to develop, as much as possible, non-drug strategies to cope with migraine, such as rest, relaxation, regular routines and exercise. If tension or pressure at school or home is acting as a trigger, stress management, relaxation, biofeedback (see p. xviii), hypnotherapy (see p. xviii) or professional counselling can be effective. Developing early coping mechanisms will help your child deal effectively with migraine in the long run. As they say, an ounce of prevention is worth a pound of cure!

Diagnosis and Management of Migraine

Proper diagnosis of migraine is an important first step in taking control of your disorder. Many people (as many as 60 percent of sufferers) have never sought medical advice for their disorder and as many as 45 percent lapse from physician care.

The next step to managing this disorder is to learn as much as possible about it, about your triggers (whether they are dietary, hormonal or stress- or environment-related) and to take steps to change your lifestyle.

Diagnosing Migraine

First and foremost, managing migraine is about obtaining a diagnosis from a physician. According to a recent study, only 50 percent of migraine sufferers have actually been diagnosed and only 34 percent regularly consult a physician.

In 1988, the International Headache Society developed guidelines that considerably improved the diagnosis of migraine. Their diagnostic criteria for migraine included attacks lasting 4 to 72 hours, and some combination of the following symptoms:

* One-sided moderate to severe throbbing pain aggravated by movement;
* Nausea or vomiting;
* Sensitivity to light and sound; and
* Visual or sensory disturbances referred to as aura.

Other key headache syndromes were also identified, including rebound headache and cluster headache. See p. x for more information on these types of headache.

Warning signs and symptoms

Many people actually experience symptoms and do not realise that they could be part of migraine. These should be checked by a physician. In addition to the more easily recognised symptoms mentioned above, many people feel more subtle signs and symptoms with their attacks. These may be experienced prior to, as well as during, an attack and can include:

- Dizziness;
- General discomfort in the stomach and/or abdominal area;
- Depression, irritability, tension and/or other alteration in mood and outlook, sometimes with a feeling of detachment;
- Inability to concentrate;
- Sensitivity to light and sound;
- Feelings of extreme well-being with uncommon energy, vigour and a feeling of excitement preceding the attack;
- Excessive yawning;
- Unusual hunger, desire for snacks, especially sweets;
- Overtalkativeness or difficulty forming words, recalling words and incidents;
- Pain or numbness in neck and shoulder areas;
- Trembling;
- Patches or blotchy areas on skin, which looks like a rash;
- Unusual paleness or pallor (especially true with children); and
- Increase in weight, perhaps along with swelling in fingers and hands, waist, breasts, ankles or legs, or an increase in frequency and volume of urination.

These warning signs and symptoms are most frequently noted by physicians and those who suffer from migraine, and are sometimes called symptoms of the 'prodrome' or aura. Individuals have suggested others that are peculiar to them. As with the more easily recognised symptoms of migraine, not everyone experiences all of these symptoms. When you discuss your migraine with your physician, it may help if you list the symptoms that refer specifically to you.

Triggers

A trigger is any internal or external influence that activates or aggravates a migraine attack. Most people find that a combination of triggers brings on an attack. Because people afflicted with migraine are sensitive to these influences, it is important to identify triggers and reduce or eliminate their impact as much as possible. It is also important to remember that triggers in and of themselves are not the cause of migraine and that migraine is a complicated biological disorder.

If you can readily identify your triggers, you will find it much easier to manage your migraine attacks. You can eliminate or avoid some triggers, reduce others, and brace for those over which you have no control. While some triggers, such as weather, are not controllable, they often work in combination with those that are controllable, such as food. For this reason, simply being aware of them will help you to manage your migraine.

Keeping a diary will help you to isolate your triggers. If you document your migraine attacks over a period of several months, you will probably notice that there is a pattern to your attacks. You should track the following items:

- Frequency of attacks
- Duration of attacks
- What the attacks felt like
- What made the pain worse and what made it better
- What other symptoms (nausea, vomiting, sensitivity to sound, light, etc.) you experienced
- What potential triggers (food, hormones, weather, stress, etc.) you were exposed to 24 to 48 hours in advance of an attack
- What medications or treatments you took and how they worked

Remember, though, that your triggers can change throughout life. Always be on the lookout for new ones and be open to the possibility that you may outgrow others.

The following list of triggers includes those that are most commonly known. Not all migraineurs will be affected by these triggers. Finding what is specific to you and avoiding or managing your triggers is the key. The five most common migraine triggers are:

Hormonal cycles or changes
- puberty
- menstruation
- birth control pills
- hormone replacement therapy
- peri-menopause

Changes in daily routine
- missing a meal
- sleeping more or less than usual

Stress
- experiencing an episode of emotional stress
- resting after an emotionally stressful period

Weather and environment
- changes in barometric pressure
- cigarette smoke (first and second-hand)

Dietary
- caffeine (coffee, tea, soft drinks) and, especially, caffeine withdrawal

- chocolate in any form
- fruits, especially citrus: oranges, lemons, limes, grapefruit, fermented dry fruits (raisins, figs, etc.), banana-peel extract, red plums, papaya and passion fruit
- beverages: beer, coloured alcohol and wine (especially red, port, sherry, sweet white), dark rum, whisky and brandy
- dairy products: cultured dairy products, such as soured cream and buttermilk; chocolate milk; acidophilus milk; aged cheese: Boursault, Brie, Camembert, Cheddar, Gouda, Gruyère, mozzarella, Parmesan, Emmental, Provolone, Romano, Roquefort and Stilton
- food additives: Aspartame – NutraSweet; MSG: Accent, ajinomoto, Chinese seasoning, flavourings (including natural), glutacyl, glutavene, hydrolysed plant protein, hydrolysed vegetable protein, kombo extract, mei-jing, RL-50, subu, vestin, wei-jing and Zest
- nuts: peanuts
- seeds: sesame, sunflower and pumpkin
- beans and vegetables: beans (butter, cannellini, broad, pinto, chick pea, lentils, green), mange tout, chilli peppers, pickles, olives, onions, garlic, peas and tomatoes
- miscellaneous: brewer's yeast
- meat, fish, poultry: chicken and beef organ meats (liver and kidney), salted or dried fish (herring, cod), fermented sausage, bacon and processed meats (sodium nitrate)

Hint: Always read the labels of prepared foods, as many of these products contain additives such as MSG that may trigger a migraine attack. For a more detailed discussion of how to manage dietary triggers, see p. xix.

Managing Migraine

After obtaining a diagnosis, you should take the following important steps in managing your migraine:

- identify your triggers by keeping a diary (see p. xxiii);
- keep a record of your triggers, as they can change over your lifetime;
- optimise physical health by maintaining a healthy diet, exercising, keeping a regular sleep regime and taking medications correctly;
- optimise mental health and learn ways to manage the stress in your life;
- consult regularly with your physician regarding treatment options; and
- obtain up-to-date information from your physician or The Migraine Action Association or The Migraine Trust (see p. 126).

Medication

When you discuss treatment options with your doctor, be aware that there are two basic types of migraine medication: symptomatic and preventive.

Symptomatic medications are taken to relieve the symptoms of an attack once it's in progress. These medications are usually more effective when they are taken in the early stages of the attack. The most common types of symptomatic medications that are available over the counter are acetylsalicylic acid (ASA), acetaminophen and ibuprofen.

Many symptomatic medications are currently available with a prescription, including a class of drugs called triptans. Triptan medications are known to the medical community as 5-HT (serotonin) receptor agonists. These medications work on the mechanism of migraine and relieve symptoms associated with migraine, such as headache pain, nausea/vomiting and sensitivity to light and sound. Triptan medications narrow (constrict) blood vessels in the head that expand (dilate) during a migraine attack. They are also thought to reduce the release of substances that cause blood vessels to become inflamed and to reduce transmission of pain impulses to the brain.

Preventive medications are taken daily to prevent or reduce the number of migraine attacks. Unlike symptomatic medications, they are not pain relievers. They work for many sufferers by correcting the underlying imbalances within the body believed to cause migraine. All preventive medications should be taken exactly as prescribed. They take time to start working, so before their effectiveness is evaluated, they should be given at least two months to start to work.

Preventive drugs include beta-blockers; calcium channel blockers; anti-depressants; monoamine-oxidase inhibitors (MAOIs); antiserotonin agents; anti-inflammatory agents and anti-convulsants.

If you are interested in knowing more about these medications, consult your physician.

Complementary Therapies

A broad range of treatments for migraine do not fall within the category of conventional medicine. These include:

- biobehavioural treatment, such as biofeedback;
- relaxation therapy and cognitive-behavioural therapy;
- bodywork or manipulation, such as chiropractic, massage and acupuncture; and
- vitamin, mineral or herbal therapies, such as riboflavin, magnesium and feverfew.

These therapies are considered 'complementary,' or 'non-pharmacological,' and for many play an important role in prevention and empowerment of the sufferer. (Many migraineurs often feel powerless over their disorder and become frustrated or angry at the lack of validation from medical professionals, family members, employers or friends.) These approaches are particularly useful when conventional treatment is inadequate, not tolerated or contra-indicated. The appropriateness of using such therapies is based on availability and cost, and the motivation and commitment of the individual seeking treatment.

In seeking treatment, it is always important to get an initial diagnosis (see p. xiii) and follow-up from a doctor. It is also important to return to a physician if there is a change in symptoms and before beginning new therapies. Beware of therapists who will not allow you to see anyone else at the same time or who have costly 'miracle cures.' Ask practitioners about their qualifications and whether their area of speciality is regulated by a professional organisation. Ask them about the theory behind their method and talk to others who have undergone the same therapy.

Biofeedback allows you to learn to alter your physiological responses at will. Machines provide feedback about biological responses in the body, such as the contraction of scalp muscles and the circulation and temperature of the hands or temple area. This information is then translated into a display – an audio tone or visual representation – that is 'fed back' to the patient.

Relaxation therapy develops long-term skills for the prevention of migraine. Different methods include muscle relaxation, breathing exercises and directed imagery. Relaxation therapy is often combined with biofeedback.

Cognitive-behavioural therapy (CBT) helps migraine sufferers identify stressful circumstances and employ effective strategies for coping. Individuals identify and modify negative responses that may trigger or aggravate migraine. CBT may also help to limit the negative psychological consequences of chronic pain, such as depression and disability. Similarly, **hypnotherapy** reduces distressing sensory input, which can act as triggers or aggravators of migraine.

Chiropractic may relieve some migraine attacks. Too much or too little movement in the cervical or neck region can cause muscle spasms around the neck, which may lead to a migraine attack. Manipulation, exercise and physical therapy improve motion and can alleviate pain.

Massage has sedative and invigorating effects, increases range of motion, improves muscle tone and stimulates the release of endorphins, the body's natural painkillers. By massaging trigger points at the top of the neck and base of the skull, the tension associated with chronic pain may be relieved.

Acupuncture, a traditional Chinese medicine that uses needles to restore the balance of energy, is believed to block the transmission of pain and stimulate the release of endorphins.

Riboflavin* or Vitamin B2 (400 mg) as well as **magnesium*** (400–600 mg) may help to reduce the frequency and severity of migraine if taken on a daily basis.

Feverfew*, which comes from a plant belonging to the chrysanthemum family, may also help migraine sufferers. It is believed to work by reducing the release of a chemical closely linked to migraine; by inhibiting the secretion of prostaglandin, a substance involved in inflammation; and by stabilising blood vessels, making them less sensitive to the release of chemicals.

* Always check with your doctor if you are planning to use riboflavin, feverfew or magnesium.

Managing Dietary Triggers

While there is no known cure for migraines, understanding your triggers can help you take charge of your attacks so that you can get your life back. Not all people are affected by food triggers – but those who are affected will find that managing them will ensure that you lead a life in which *you* are in control; identifying and avoiding your food triggers will help give you back a measure of control over your life.

Arguably, one of the most modifiable factors in migraine management is diet. While controversy remains around the relationship between the frequency and severity of migraines and the consumption of certain foods and substances, like additives and preservatives, contained in foods, there is little doubt that diet may play a significant role in triggering, or initiating, migraine. Adjusting your diet, *not* restricting your diet, will give you greater control over your attacks. Adjusting your diet, while ensuring that you are consuming an adequate amount of nutrients, will help you manage your migraine attacks, and stay healthy, whether you experience these headaches frequently or intermittently.

A substantial number of migraine sufferers experience an attack shortly after (or within 24 to 48 hours) consuming a particular food or combination of foods. As mentioned above, identifying your food triggers and then avoiding them in your diet is an important step in migraine management; in your taking back control. In this section, we will discuss food triggers, and how to identify them; migraines and MSG; and how to track your food triggers by keeping a trigger diary.

The information in the following pages should help you to recognise the foods, as well as the chemicals and additives contained in foods, that may trigger your migraines. Then turn to the recipe section for meal planning suggestions that will have you eating delicious foods that should not trigger an attack. You will soon recognise that you are not at the mercy of your migraines, and that you have, at your fingertips, and in your kitchen, an arsenal with which to fight them.

It is important to note that the actual foods you eat are not necessarily the only triggers to your migraines; that is, they are usually collaborating with some of your other dietary habits, for example, skipping meals, fasting or delaying meals. Moreover, dietary triggers may also be interacting with other triggers, as discussed on page xv – environmental, stress, medication-related or hormonal.

Food Trigger or Food Allergy?

A food trigger is not a food allergy; a food allergy is an immune-system response to a protein contained in food. While some researchers believe that food allergies do cause headaches, most believe that they in themselves play no role in causing headache, but that the substances contained within some foods trigger the headache by changing the body's neurochemical balance, for example by altering the balance of the neurotransmitter (a kind of chemical messenger) serotonin, or by narrowing and then expanding blood vessels in the brain. It is important to note that since food allergies do not appear to cause migraines, allergy testing won't get you any further ahead in identifying your dietary triggers.

Anatomy of a Food Trigger

You eat a sausage roll for lunch or go to your favourite Chinese restaurant for dinner, and within 24 hours, you suffer a debilitating migraine attack. Why does this happen? According to the *Canadian Medical Association Journal*, "[the] ingestion of foods containing nitrites, aspartame or monosodium glutamate, and the cumulative effect of eating foods with a high content of neurotransmitter precursors, such as tyramine, tyrosine and phenylalanine, are associated with the precipitation of migraine headache. . . ." (CMAJ: 1997; 156(9)). Sausage rolls, and other smoked or preserved meats, like luncheon meats, ham, bacon and hot dogs, contain nitrites; and Chinese food is notorious for containing the flavour enhancer monosodium glutamate (see p. xxii); both these substances are implicated in the triggering of migraine attacks. They cause neurological disturbances that make the blood vessels in the brain swell, which further causes them to press on the surrounding nerves, which may trigger an attack.

Many foods that initiate migraine attacks contain substances, called vasoactive amines, that affect the body's blood vessels, especially those that supply blood to the brain. Vasoactive amines widen or narrow the blood vessels in the brain, which is responsible for the pain of the migraine headache. Food sources include any items that have been fermented; for example, ripened cheeses; these foods contain a substance known as tyramine. Tyramine can also be found in red organ meats (such as beef and chicken liver) and any pickled products.

Another amine implicated in the cause of migraines is phenylethlamine, a food source of which is chocolate in any form. Citrus fruits and their juices, also on the list of foods for some migraineurs to avoid, contain another headache-producing amine, synephrine.

Common sources of amine-containing foods include: fruits (avocado, banana, citrus fruits, pineapple, red-skinned fruits); vegetables (spinach, aubergine, skin of potatoes and tomatoes); beverages (dark alcoholic drinks, tea); dairy products (ripened cheeses, buttermilk, yogurt, soured cream); herbs and spices; and cured, pickled or marinated products. It is important to note that the amount of amine may be very slight and, in many cases, is not enough to trigger an attack.

The Migraineur's Storecupboard

A variety of foods and food additives are known to trigger migraine attacks (see p. xv for a list of the common dietary triggers), but it is important to note that not all these foods act as triggers to all migraineurs; people who are sensitive to one food may, in fact, be able to eat it in small quantities if they have managed to control other triggers. As mentioned earlier, food triggers often do not act alone, but in collaboration with other triggers (see p. xiv).

Profiles of the usual suspects

Caffeine: Caffeine – or caffeine withdrawal – is often a trigger. In some cases, the ingestion of excessive amounts as part of a medication may be the culprit. Coffee and tea are common trigger foods, but remember that caffeine is also present in chocolate and soft drinks.

Chocolate: The more concentrated the chocolate is, the more likely it is to trigger a migraine. Unsweetened and bitter chocolate, for example, are the most concentrated. Some people can consume milk chocolate or white chocolate in modest amounts, and not risk suffering a migraine attack.

So, what's a chocoholic to do? Turn to the recipes section, and try Carob Chip Cookies (p. 109) or No-Bake Carob-Oatmeal Macaroons (p. 110). These delectable 'chocolate' treats will make even the most hardened chocoholic's mouth water.

Fruits: The most common triggers in this category are citrus fruits (lemons, limes, oranges and grapefruit). Some people can eat small quantities of these fruits and not suffer a migraine attack. Other food triggers in this category include: papaya, mangoes, kiwi, pineapple, plums, avocado and dried fruits that contain preservatives, for example, raisins, figs and dates. These foods also contain vasoactive amines, which, as mentioned earlier, affect the blood vessels that supply blood to the brain.

Try the Herb and Cherry Tabbouleh (p. 77) or the Roasted Pears with Minted Custard (p. 91) for some fruity delights.

Alcohol: Alcoholic beverages can dilate blood vessels in the brain and for some trigger migraine attacks. Red wine and other 'coloured' alcoholic beverages, like dark rum, brandy, sherry, port and whisky, are more common culprits in triggering migraine attacks; the yeast contained in beer is also often implicated. Some migraineurs can tolerate white wine and other light-coloured alcoholic drinks (vodka, for example), taken in modest amounts. It is important to remember that alcohol might negatively interact with medication you are taking for migraine as well as dehydrate you.

If you enjoy cooking with red wine, and need a substitute for this potential food trigger, use vodka or white wine instead; try the Filo-Wrapped Chicken with Mushrooms and Spinach in Citron Vodka Sauce (p. 45), or the Scallops with White Wine and Tarragon Sauce (p. 64).

For a soothing, non-alcoholic drink, with medicinal qualities, try the Migraine Mellower (p. 116).

Dairy products: Cultured or fermented dairy products can be powerful triggers for some. Sources include yogurt and soured cream, chocolate milk, buttermilk, cultured butter, acidophilus milk and aged cheeses like Boursault, Brie, Camembert, Cheddar, Gouda, Gruyère, mozzarella, Parmesan, Emmental, Provolone, Romano, Roquefort and Stilton. If you want to use cheese in a recipe, try unaged or mild cheeses, like cottage cheese, goats' cheese and yogurt made from skimmed milk. Eggs are also a safe food choice, unlikely to trigger an attack. Also note that it is safe to drink skimmed milk.

If you find yourself yearning for cheese, try the delicious Warm Goats' Cheese Salad with Grilled Vegetables (p. 20), the Toasted Creamy Goats' Cheese with Onion Confit (p. 22) or the marvellous Vegetable and Cheese Lasagne (p. 32).

Monosodium glutamate (MSG): This substance can be a powerful migraine trigger. Common sources include packet foods, powdered or canned soups, stock cubes, frozen ready-meals and snack foods. There are also a number of hidden sources of MSG. Indeed, even if we carefully read food labels, and decide the ingredients are 'safe', we are frequently unaware of the MSG that is hidden in some other substance that is listed. MSG often lurks in the guise of polysyllabic, indecipherable ingredients.

Here is a list of ingredients that always contain MSG:

Monosodium glutamate	Hydrolysed protein
Sodium caseinate	Yeast extract
Yeast nutrient	Autolysed yeast
Textured protein	Yeast food
Calcium caseinate	Hydrolysed oat flour

Artificial sweeteners: These substances, especially aspartame (NutraSweet; Equal) have been found to trigger migraine attacks in some people. Aspartame is frequently used in diet soft drinks and in sugarless chewing gum. Other artificial sweeteners, such as cyclamate (Sugar Twin) and sucralose (Splenda) do not appear to trigger migraine attacks.

Nuts and seeds: If you are predisposed to migraines, peanuts (and peanut butter), and seeds, such as sesame, sunflower and pumpkin seeds, can be a trigger and may induce an attack. We include avocadoes in this category, although people usually think of them as a fruit.

Beans and vegetables: Onions and tomatoes (although these are considered by some to be a fruit) are often identified as migraine triggers. Other triggers in this category include: chilli peppers, beans (butter, cannellini, broad, pinto, chick pea, lentils, green), mange tout and lentils. Olives, pickles and sauerkraut have also been identified as possible culprits.

Delight in the fragrance and flavours of Steamed Basmati Rice with Crisp Potatoes, Sumac and Cumin (p. 76), Bulgur and Green Bean Salad with Herbed Vinaigrette (p. 78) or Charred Courgettes with Herbs, Garlic and Ricotta (p. 73).

Breads and yeast-raised baked goods: These foods contain yeast, which may trigger a migraine attack. Commercially prepared breads appear to present less of a problem to migraineurs than their hot, fresh homemade counterparts. Before eating your beautiful homemade bread, let it sit for a while to cool; this may reduce its effect as a migraine trigger.

Try the Irish Scones (p. 84) or the Corn Bread (p. 86) for delicious breads that will not trigger a migraine attack.

Meat, poultry and fish: Fresh beef, poultry and fish are not implicated as migraine triggers, but organ meats, such as kidney and liver, may trigger an attack. Also in this category are processed or smoked meats, which contain nitrites, including hot dogs, luncheon meats, ham, bacon and sausage; and smoked, salted or pickled fish.

Sample the Curried Chicken with Peaches and Coconut (p. 38), the Roast Duck with Spiced Honey (p. 44) or the Fresh Tuna with Maple Mustard Sauce and Coriander Oil (p. 53) as succulent main courses.

Miscellaneous: Although it seems rare, some people report suffering migraine attacks after consuming products containing food colourings and dyes, for example, as used in confectionary, powdered drinks, gelatine desserts; and after consuming vinegar, as contained in ketchup, mayonnaise and salad dressings.

Skipping Meals Can Trigger an Attack

If you are predisposed to migraines, don't skip meals, especially breakfast! A low blood sugar level caused by skipping meals, or other dietary practices, like irregular mealtimes or weight-loss diets, often trigger migraine attacks. Skipping breakfast is an especially dangerous practice if you're a migraineur; blood sugar levels are particularly low in the morning, and skipping breakfast can therefore trigger a headache later in the day. (Turn to the recipe section of the book and let yourself be tempted by the Pancakes, p. 88, or the Apple Pancakes, p. 89.)

To keep your blood sugar levels stable during the day, eat a number of small meals at regular intervals, rather than two or three large meals. Consume these meals no more than four or five hours apart. Refer to the recipe section of the book for snacks and meals that will keep your blood sugar levels from dipping too low, and thus avoid suffering a migraine attack. Sample the Oatcakes (p. 2) or the Herbed Pitta Crisps (p. 3) for a migraine-free dietary pick-me-up.

Tracking the Culprits: Your Food Trigger Diary

Once you've examined the contents of your storecupboard and fridge, and thought carefully about your food consumption patterns and all your triggers, you're well on the way to identifying the foods and beverages that may be responsible for triggering your migraine attacks. A diary in which you diligently track all the foods you eat each day will help you further identify the items to steer clear of if you want to avoid an attack.

In a survey undertaken recently GPs identified keeping a diary as the single most helpful thing a migraine patient could do to help them to understand their condition and obtain appropriate treatment.

Keeping a diary will help you determine your 'trigger threshold' – the number of triggers you can be exposed to before experiencing an attack. For example, you may drink a cup of coffee and not end up in the grips of a migraine; but you may find that drinking a second cup, skipping a meal and being overtired or overstressed will push you over the threshold, and you will experience a migraine attack.

In your diary, record:
- the food (or beverage) you consumed (include alcoholic beverages and those containing caffeine);

- the amount you consumed; and
- the time you consumed it. (Note that it may take your body 24 to 48 hours to react to a trigger.)

Also record any headaches you experience, and note:
- date;
- time of day;
- location of head pain (behind the eyes; squeezing head like a band; pounding on either side of head; at top of head, radiating down sides);
- duration;
- frequency;
- severity; and
- other symptoms (vomiting, nausea, sensitivity to light and sound).

You should also document other triggers such as weather, stress, hormonal fluctuations and so on, since, as mentioned earlier, food triggers often work with other trigger accomplices.

Testing your triggers

As a pattern emerges, you may notice a correlation between your consumption of a food or beverage and the incidence and severity of your migraine attacks. Add these to your food triggers list and avoid eating them; find delicious substitutes in the recipe section of this book.

Avoid in your diet the triggers identified in your diary, then re-introduce each of your 'forbidden' foods. If you find you experience no symptoms when the food is not included in your diet, and the symptoms reappear when the food is re-introduced, this food may be one of those triggering your migraine attack.

Documenting the foods and beverages you consume is not a complicated task, and is well worth the effort in helping you get your life back.

For more information on how to identify your personal triggers contact The Migraine Action Association or The Migraine Trust (see page 126 for Resources Directory).

Checklist for avoiding migraines

1. *Know* your food triggers: keep a list of them at hand, perhaps on the fridge door, where you can see them each time you're tempted to reach for that chocolate ice cream or a hunk of Cheddar.
2. *Document* the foods you eat each day, in a migraine diary, in order to identify the substances that may be initiating your migraine attacks.
3. *Note* all your triggers, including your sleep patterns, changes in weather, hormonal fluctuations, and the incidence of stressful events.
4. *Read* food labels when you're food shopping, to make sure trigger ingredients are not contained in the food item you are about to purchase. And be aware of hidden food triggers.
5. *Enjoy* the delectable, mouthwatering, migraine-free recipes in this book.

The Last Word. . . .

It is a challenge living comfortably with migraine; in fact, the idea that one can live comfortably with these often debilitating headaches may appear to be absurd, an impossibility. However, by controlling the modifiable factors in your daily life, by managing your triggers and discussing treatment options with your doctor, you can regain control of your life.

You may wonder how on earth you're going to find anything to eat or how you're ever going to plan a meal, since everything you enjoy seems to be a potential trigger. The answer is in some of the suggestions made in this section and in the recipe portion of this cookbook. Use the recipes in the following pages to prepare mouthwatering dishes that are free of widely acknowledged food triggers. You will find recipes for appetisers and snacks, soups and salads, meatless main courses, meat and poultry, fish and seafood, vegetables and side dishes, breads, desserts and baked goods, and beverages. Plan your meals using these recipes, and you will enjoy eating wonderful foods with the knowledge that you are not setting yourself up for a migraine attack.

How to Use This Cookbook

The recipes found within these pages are delicious and nutritious and range from the easy-to-create to the more sophisticated.

Wherever possible, we have attempted to minimise the number of potential food triggers contained in the recipes or we have suggested substitutions. To help you readily identify the recipes that are appropriate for you, we have included a trigger coding system for each recipe. It outlines the ten most common triggers and indicates the specific triggers that have been avoided or eliminated. For example, if a recipe contains no citrus fruit (lemon, lime, orange or grapefruit), it is ticked as being citrus-free.

Each recipe also contains a nutritional analysis and all recipes are calculated per serving size, unless otherwise indicated. Where there is a choice, the nutritional analysis is based on the smaller quantity and on the first ingredient. When ingredients are optional, they are not included in the analysis. Milk is calculated using skimmed milk unless otherwise indicated.

Note should be taken that recipe servings vary, some serve 2, others serve 4-6, 6-8 or even 10. This is to provide a range of meals for all occasions from family suppers to entertaining friends. The number of servings is given at the end of every recipe. Quantities can be scaled up or down according to your requirements.

Bon appétit!

Appetisers and Snacks

Oatcakes

Herbed Pitta Crisps

Vegetable Platter with Olive Oil Dip (Pinzimonio)

Houmous

Shiitake Perogies with Sweet Ginger Sauce

Prawn Pastries

Grilled Gravadlax with Mustard Dill Sauce

Oatcakes

These traditional Scottish oatcakes can be served warm or cold and they are delicious with cottage cheese and celery or butter and jam and are ideal for children to snack on.

125 g	medium oatmeal	4 oz
½ tsp	salt	½ tsp
½ tsp	bicarbonate of soda	½ tsp
2 tsp	oil	2 tsp
	boiling water	

Mix the oats with the salt and bicarbonate of soda, then add the oil and sufficient boiling water to make a soft dough.

Knead lightly on a floured surface, then roll out thinly into a 20 cm/8 inch circle. Cut the round into 8 wedges.

The oatcakes can either be baked in the oven on a greased baking sheet at 200°C/400°F/Gas Mark 6 for 15-20 minutes or baked in a heavy oiled frying pan.

Make sure the pan is really hot (test by dropping in a few oats which should turn brown instantly). Bake the oatcakes for 3-4 minutes on each side until lightly browned.

These oatcakes should be crisp, browned and curling up at edges. Leave to cool.

Makes 8 oatcakes.

PER SERVING (1 BISCUIT)	
Kcals	69.40
g fat	2.11
g protein	1.94
g carbohydrate	11.38

Herbed Pitta Crisps

These crunchy, flavoursome crisps are ideal for a light snack.

8	large pitta breads	8
175 g	butter, melted	6 oz
1 tsp	each dried oregano, marjoram, basil, and parsley flakes	1 tsp

Separate each pitta bread into two thin rounds.
Using scissors, cut the rounds into eight pieces each.
Combine the melted butter, oregano, marjoram, basil and parsley in a small bowl then brush all over the pitta pieces.
Place on greased baking sheets and bake at 150°C/300°F/ Gas Mark 2 for 30 minutes.
Makes 128 pitta crisps.

PER SERVING (1 PITTA CRISP)	
Kcals	30
g fat	2
g protein	trace
g carbohydrate	3

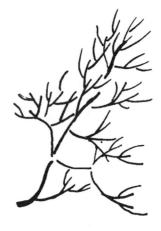

Vegetable Platter with Olive Oil Dip (Pinzimonio)

An Italian idea, this healthy, easy-to-prepare appetiser consists simply of an assortment of fresh vegetables and extra virgin olive oil.

fresh vegetables, such as carrots, cucumbers, red or yellow peppers, cherry tomatoes, fennel bulbs, and radishes, trimmed and chopped
extra virgin olive oil
salt
crusty bread (optional)
prosciutto, sliced paper thin (optional)

Arrange the vegetables on a platter. The quantity is flexible, depending on how many people you are serving. Drizzle the olive oil onto individual plates and season to taste with salt. The vegetables are then dipped into the olive oil. For additional flavour, serve with bread and prosciutto, although you'll want to avoid the latter if nitrates are a trigger for you.

Variation: Many vegetables can be served raw, but you may want to blanch some like green beans, mangetout and broccoli florets.

This recipe is FREE of the following triggers (marked ✔)

Caffeine ✔
Chocolate ✔
Citrus fruits ✔
Red wine ✔
Aged cheese ✔
MSG & Nitrates
Aspartame ✔
Nuts ✔
Onions & Garlic ✔
Yeast

Houmous

A Middle Eastern speciality, houmous is ideal served with Herbed Pitta Crisps (see p. 3) or as a vegetable dip.

(see p. 3)

400 g	can chickpeas	14 oz
75 ml	(about) hot water	3 fl oz
1	juice of large lemon	1
2	cloves garlic	2
4 tbsp	tahini	4 tbsp
	virgin olive oil	
	salt	
	chilli powder (optional)	

Drain and rinse the chickpeas. Process in a food processor, gradually adding enough of the hot water to make a purée. Add the lemon juice, garlic, tahini, about 1 tablespoon of oil and season with salt. Process until well blended and smooth. Taste and adjust seasonings, if necessary.

Scrape into a serving bowl, drizzle with more olive oil, and sprinkle with the chilli powder, if using.

Makes about 250 ml/9 fl oz.

Variation: Fresh chopped parsley and lightly toasted pine nuts can also be used as garnishes.

This recipe is FREE of the following triggers (marked ✔)

Caffeine ✔
Chocolate ✔
Citrus fruits ✔
Red wine ✔
Aged cheese ✔
MSG & Nitrates ✔
Aspartame ✔
Nuts ✔
Onions & Garlic
Yeast ✔

PER SERVING (1 TBSP)	
Kcals	59
g fat	3
g protein	2
g carbohydrate	6

Shiitake Perogies with Sweet Ginger Sauce

These dainty, vegetarian perogies make an elegant and tasty appetiser. If MSG is a trigger, make sure you use a naturally brewed soy sauce or Homemade Soy Sauce (see p. 125).

225 g	mashed potatoes (cold leftovers are perfect)	8 oz
100 g	fresh shiitake mushrooms, finely chopped (stems removed)	4 oz
1	clove garlic, crushed	1
½ tsp	fresh coriander leaves, finely chopped	½ tsp
12	wonton wrappers	12
Sweet Ginger Sauce		
2 tsp	soy sauce (naturally brewed or Homemade, p. 125)	2 tsp
1 tsp	cornflour	1 tsp
125 ml	chicken or vegetable stock (see p. 121-122)	4 fl oz
1 tsp	grated fresh ginger	1 tsp
2 tsp	sugar	2 tsp
1 tsp	butter	1 tsp

Put the mashed potatoes in a large bowl with the mushrooms, garlic and coriander and mix together. Place 1 tablespoon of this mixture on each wonton wrapper and wet the rim with water. Close and press together to seal. Boil or shallow fry dumplings over high heat for about 3 minutes or until cooked through. Set aside.

For the Sweet Ginger Sauce, combine the soy sauce and cornflour. Add to the remaining ingredients in saucepan. Bring the sauce to the boil and simmer until thickened. Serve with the Shiitake Perogies.
Serves 6.

Make Ahead: Shiitake Perogies can be prepared up to a day ahead and stored in an airtight container in the fridge. Cook perogies just before serving. The sauce can also be prepared a day or two in advance, stored in the fridge, and heated just before serving.

This recipe is FREE of the following triggers (marked ✔)

Caffeine ✔
Chocolate ✔
Citrus fruits ✔
Red wine ✔
Aged cheese ✔
MSG & Nitrates ✔
Aspartame ✔
Nuts ✔
Onions & Garlic
Yeast ✔

PER SERVING

Kcals	53
g fat	1
g protein	1
g carbohydrate	10

Right:
Cream of Spinach Soup
(page 12)

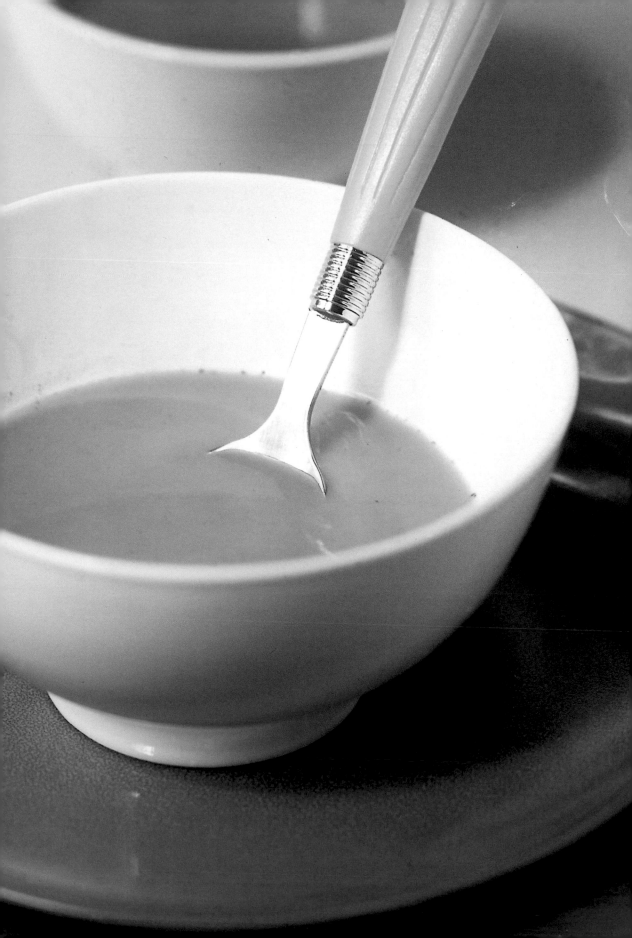

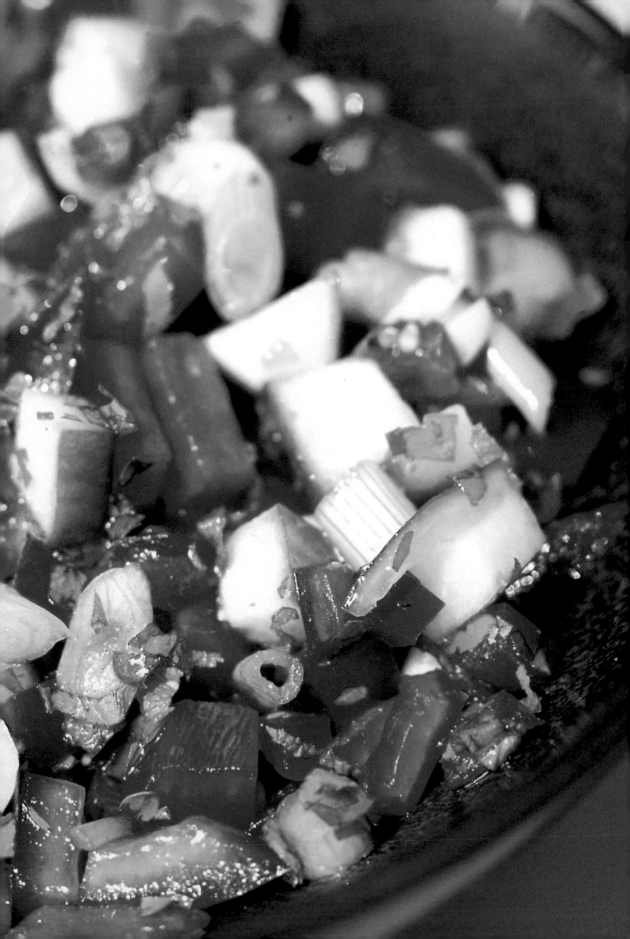

Prawn Pastries

Delicate morsels of prawn inside a lightly fried golden crust – these scrumptious appetisers will keep your guests coming back for more. If lemon juice is a trigger for you, you might consider using finely chopped lemon grass instead.

PER SERVING	
Kcals	742
g fat	38
g protein	18
g carbohydrate	82

Filling

2 tbsp	olive oil	2 tbsp
1	onion, chopped	1
2	cloves garlic, chopped	2
225 g	raw prawns, peeled, and each chopped into 3	8 oz
250 ml	water	9 fl oz
4	eggs	4
250 ml	milk	9 fl oz
2 tbsp	plain flour	2 tbsp
2 tbsp	cornflour	2 tbsp
	salt and pepper	
	lemon juice, to taste	
2 tbsp	chopped parsley	2 tbsp
pinch	nutmeg	pinch

Dough

500 ml	water	18 fl oz
500 ml	milk	18 fl oz
150 g	vegetable fat	5 oz
50 g	butter	2 oz
pinch	salt	pinch
	pepper	
300 g	plain flour	10 oz
100 g	self-raising flour	4 oz
100 g	cornflour	4 oz
50 g	fine breadcrumbs	2 oz

Left:
Middle Eastern Salad
(page 19)

Filling

Heat the olive oil in a saucepan over moderate heat.
Add the onion and garlic and fry until the onions are golden.
Add the prawns and cook for 1 minute. Add the water,
stirring until mixture comes to a boil.

Meanwhile, mix two of the eggs, the milk, flour and
cornflour in a bowl. Add to the mixture in the saucepan.
Add salt and pepper to taste, lemon juice, parsley and
nutmeg and bring to the boil. Remove from heat and leave
the mixture to cool.

Dough

Pour the water and milk into a large saucepan. Add the
vegetable fat, butter, salt and pepper to taste. Bring the
mixture to the boil. Add both flours and cornflour and mix
gradually to a paste. Remove from the heat.

Roll out the dough on a lightly floured surface to 3 mm/
1/8 inch thick. Cut into 7.5 cm/3 inch circles using round
pastry cutter. Place 1 tablespoonful of filling in the centre of
each circle, fold over to form half-moon shapes and press to
seal the dough.

Beat the two remaining eggs and brush all over the
pastries, then toss in the breadcrumbs.

Deep fry in oil heated to 190°C/375°F until golden.
Let cool and serve on platter lined with lettuce leaves.
Serves 6.

Make Ahead: The prawn filling can be prepared up to
2 days ahead and stored in the fridge. The pastries can be
assembled a day ahead, chilled, and cooked just before
serving.

Grilled Gravadlax
with Mustard Dill Sauce

The sweetly pungent dill sauce goes well with gravadlax. Some mustards contain MSG, so watch for this potential trigger – the same amount of mustard powder can often be used instead.

450 g	gravadlax, cut into 8 slices	1 lb
	extra virgin olive oil	

Mustard Dill Sauce

1 tsp	English mustard powder	1 tsp
2 tbsp	water	2 tbsp
2 tbsp	grain mustard	2 tbsp
1	egg yolk	1
1 tsp	sugar	1 tsp
100 ml	vegetable oil	4 fl oz
2 tbsp	chopped fresh dill	2 tbsp
	dill sprigs	

For the Mustard Dill Sauce, dissolve the mustard powder in the water in a small bowl. Add the grain mustard, egg yolk and sugar. Gradually whisk in the oil, then add the chopped dill.

Lightly oil the gravadlax and place in a preheated ridged cast iron pan. Cook for 1-2 minutes on each side or until lightly browned.

Place two slices of gravadlax on individual plates and spoon some mustard sauce around it. Garnish with sprigs of fresh dill.

Serves 4.

PER SERVING	
Kcals	416
g fat	36
g protein	21
g carbohydrate	2

Soups and Salads

Cream of Mushroom Soup

Cream of Spinach Soup

Pumpkin Bisque

Vichyssoise

Curried Winter Vegetable Soup

Easy Fish Chowder

Roasted Potato Salad

Grated Root Vegetable Salad with Roasted Apple Dressing

Middle Eastern Salad

Warm Goats' Cheese Salad with Grilled Vegetables

Toasted Creamy Goats' Cheese with Onion Confit

Grilled Portobello Mushrooms with Goats' Cheese and Rocket

Black-Eyed Bean Salad with Peppers

Curried Chicken and Rice Salad with Almonds

Warm Spinach Salad with Prawns

Cream of Mushroom Soup

An earthy and satisfying beginning to an autumn or winter meal. The recipe calls for a small amount of onion, but this ingredient can be omitted if it is a trigger for you.

25 g	butter	1 oz
1 tsp	chopped onion	1 tsp
100 g	mushrooms, chopped	4 oz
3 tbsp	plain flour	3 tbsp
1 tsp	salt	1 tsp
pinch	pepper	pinch
500 ml	chicken stock (see p. 122)	18 fl oz
500 ml	milk	18 fl oz

Melt the butter in a saucepan over moderate heat and fry the onion and mushrooms until softened. Blend in the flour and add salt and pepper. Cook, stirring for 2 minutes. Gradually stir in chicken stock and milk. Heat until steaming and serve immediately.
Serves 4.

This recipe is FREE of the following triggers (marked ✔)

Caffeine ✓
Chocolate ✓
Citrus fruits ✓
Red wine ✓
Aged cheese ✓
MSG & Nitrates ✓
Aspartame ✓
Nuts ✓
Onions & Garlic
Yeast ✓

PER SERVING	
Kcals	148
g fat	8
g protein	6
g carbohydrate	13

Cream of Spinach Soup

This soup is rich but light and tastes as fresh as spinach itself.

1 litre	chicken stock (see p. 122)	1¾ pints
200 g	fresh spinach, chopped	7 oz
1	onion, sliced (omit if onion is trigger)	1
100 ml	single cream	4 fl oz
	salt and pepper	
	fresh parsley for garnish	

Pour the chicken stock in to a large saucepan, bring to the boil, and add the spinach and onion. Reduce the heat and simmer for about 10 minutes.

Let the soup cool slightly, then pour into a blender and process until smooth. Return the mixture to the saucepan and heat through. Add the cream, salt and pepper to taste and heat until hot. Serve garnished with chopped parsley.
Serves 4.

This recipe is FREE of the following triggers (marked ✔)

Caffeine ✔
Chocolate ✔
Citrus fruits ✔
Red wine ✔
Aged cheese ✔
MSG & Nitrates ✔
Aspartame ✔
Nuts ✔
Onions & Garlic
Yeast ✔

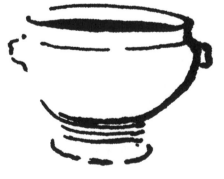

PER SERVING	
Kcals	112
g fat	8
g protein	4
g carbohydrate	6

Pumpkin Bisque

This smooth, full-flavoured soup is a perfect make-ahead first course for an autumn dinner party. It also freezes well and can be reheated in the microwave.

25 g	butter	1 oz
2	leeks (white part), thinly sliced	2
100 g	each diced carrot and parsnip	4 oz
450 g	pumpkin flesh	1 lb
1.25 litres	chicken stock (see p. 122)	2¼ pints
1 tsp	dried thyme	1 tsp
½ tsp	salt	½ tsp
¼ tsp	pepper	¼ tsp
pinch	chilli flakes (optional)	pinch
150 ml	milk	¼ pint
2 tbsp	snipped chives	2 tbsp

Melt the butter in a large saucepan over low heat. Add the leeks, carrots, parsnips and pumpkin, and cook for about 10 minutes, until softened.

Stir in the stock, thyme, salt, pepper, and chilli flakes, if using.

Bring to the boil, reduce the heat, cover and simmer for 10 minutes or until the vegetables are very soft.

Allow to cool slightly then purée in batches in a blender or food processor, until smooth. Return to the saucepan. Stir in the milk and heat through gently but do not boil. Taste and adjust seasoning. Serve sprinkled with chives.

Serves 8.

PER SERVING	
Kcals	108
g fat	4
g protein	3
g carbohydrate	15

Vichyssoise

This potato and leek soup is best served very cold.
The potatoes provide a rich thickness and the leeks a
delicate flavour. If onions are a trigger, you might want to
skip this because leeks and chives are in the same family
of vegetables.

15 g	butter	½ oz
4	leeks, finely sliced	4
1	large onion, finely sliced	1
4	medium potatoes, peeled and diced	4
500 ml	chicken stock (see p. 122)	18 fl oz
	salt and pepper	
150 ml	cream	¼ pint
	chives or parsley	

Melt the butter in a saucepan over moderate heat. Add the
leeks and onions and fry until softened but not brown.
Add the diced potatoes and chicken stock, and season with
salt and pepper. Simmer for about 30 minutes or until the
potatoes are tender.

Cool slightly then purée in a blender or food processor
until smooth.

Pour into a bowl, cover and chill in the fridge for at least
2 hours. Stir in the cream.

Adjust the seasoning if necessary, and ladle the soup into
chilled bowls. Sprinkle with chives or chopped parsley
before serving.

Serves 4.

**This recipe is FREE of the
following triggers
(marked ✔)**

Caffeine ✔
Chocolate ✔
Citrus fruits ✔
Red wine ✔
Aged cheese ✔
MSG & Nitrates ✔
Aspartame ✔
Nuts ✔
Onions & Garlic
Yeast ✔

PER SERVING	
Kcals	259
g fat	7
g protein	6
g carbohydrate	43

Curried Winter Vegetable Soup

This hearty soup can be adapted to meet specific dietary needs. For a little variety, add some chopped kale or leftover lettuce and serve with toasted French bread. It's great served with warm scones (see Healthy Scones on p. 83).

25 g	butter	1 oz
1 tsp	each cumin, curry powder, rosemary, pepper and sage	1 tsp
4 to 6	cloves garlic, crushed	4 to 6
1	large leek, chopped	1
1 litre	chicken or vegetable stock (see p. 122 and 121)	1¾ pints
250 ml	water	9 fl oz
1	medium swede, peeled and cubed	1
200 g	split lentils (red and/or yellow)	7 oz
2	medium sweet potatoes, peeled and diced	2
1	medium waxy potato, peeled and diced	1
2	medium carrots, peeled and sliced	2
1	medium parsnip, peeled and sliced	1
50 ml	coconut milk (or milk)	2 fl oz
2 tbsp	finely chopped coriander or parsley	2 tbsp

Melt the butter in a large saucepan. Stir in the cumin, curry powder, rosemary, pepper and sage. Add the garlic and leek. Cook over a low heat, for 2-5 minutes or until the leek is tender. Add the stock, water, swede and lentils. Bring to the boil slowly, then reduce the heat, cover and simmer for 10 minutes. Add the potatoes, carrots and parsnip.

Simmer, covered, for 25-40 minutes or until potatoes, carrots and parsnips are tender. Remove from heat and allow to cool slightly until all the bubbling has stopped. Mash roughly with a potato masher. Stir in the coconut milk or milk, coriander or parsley. Return to the heat briefly to warm through, then serve.

Serves 6-8.

Variations: These are endless as any vegetable can easily be added or substituted in this recipe. Cooked meat can also be added. Pearl barley can be used instead of lentils, but more cooking time should be allowed.

PER SERVING	
Kcals	211
g fat	3
g protein	9
g carbohydrate	37

Easy Fish Chowder

Serve this nutritious chowder with crusty bread.

25 g	butter	1 oz
4	medium potatoes, diced	4
2-3	thinly sliced celery stalks	2-3
150 g	grated carrot	5 oz
1 tsp	rosemary	1 tsp
	salt and pepper	
225 g	fish fillets (cod, haddock, or any firm white fish), or 142 g/5 oz can baby clams (with juice)	8 oz
500 ml	evaporated milk	18 fl oz

Melt the butter in a large saucepan over moderate heat. Add the potatoes, celery and carrot and fry until softened. Cover with water (or clam juice, if using), and add the rosemary and salt and pepper to taste. Simmer until tender.

Add the fish, cut into pieces, and simmer until the fish flakes easily when tested with fork. Stir in the milk and heat through without boiling. Taste and adjust seasoning before serving.

Serves 4.

PER SERVING	
Kcals	392
g fat	16
g protein	23
g carbohydrate	39

Roasted Potato Salad

A fresh and satisfying alternative to your usual potato salad. Serve with a loaf of fresh, crusty bread.

1	whole garlic head	1
1 tbsp	(approx.) olive oil	1 tbsp
	salt and pepper	
1 kg	potatoes, scrubbed and cut into chunks	2 lb 4 oz
1	red pepper	1
1	small red onion, chopped	1

Balsamic Vinaigrette

4 tbsp	olive oil	4 tbsp
2 tbsp	balsamic vinegar (or cider vinegar plus 2 tbsp brown sugar)	2 tbsp
1 tsp	Dijon mustard (or ½ tsp English mustard powder, if MSG is a trigger)	1 tsp
1 tsp	fresh thyme	1 tsp
pinch	each cayenne, salt and pepper	pinch

   Cut 1 cm/½ inch off the top of the garlic head and place in small baking dish. Drizzle with some oil and season with salt and pepper. Cover with foil and bake 150°C/300°F/Gas Mark 2 for 1½ hours, or until tender when squeezed. Leave to cool.
   Heat 1 tbsp oil in a roasting pan at 220°C/425°F/Gas Mark 7 until hot. Add the potatoes and toss to coat. Roast for 35 minutes or until soft and golden, turning often.
   For the vinaigrette, whisk all the ingredients together in a small bowl.
   Squeeze the roasted garlic pulp into a serving bowl. Add the potatoes, red pepper, onion and vinaigrette. Toss together then taste and adjust the seasoning. Serve warm or at room temperature.
   Serves 4-6.

PER SERVING (WHEN RECIPE SERVES 6)	
Kcals	234
g fat	10
g protein	4
g carbohydrate	32

Grated Root Vegetable Salad with Roasted Apple Dressing

The unusual dressing gives this salad an exceptional flavour.

2	Granny Smith apples, peeled and cored	2
	olive oil, as needed	
	sea salt	
2	medium beetroot, peeled	2
2	parsnips, peeled	2
1	carrot, peeled	1
1	celeriac, peeled	1
1	head soft round lettuce	1

Dressing
Peel and core the apples and arrange neatly in lightly oiled frying pan.

Season with sea salt, if desired, and cook over moderately high heat, turning occasionally, until tender and golden (do not allow to burn).

Transfer the cooked apples to a food processor and process until smooth. Gradually pour in olive oil, until the dressing is creamy.

Salad
Grate the vegetables, keeping each vegetable separate and covered until ready to serve.

Spread some apple dressing on individual salad plates and arrange small mounds of grated vegetables around the rim. Place lettuce leaves in the centre of each plate and drizzle over the remaining dressing.

Serves 4.

Kitchen Pointer: Remember to grate the vegetables as thinly as possible using a mandolin with the julienne attachment, or other favourite vegetable grater.

Make ahead: The apple dressing can be prepared earlier in the day and chilled.

This recipe is FREE of the following triggers (marked ✔)

Caffeine ✔
Chocolate ✔
Citrus fruits ✔
Red wine ✔
Aged cheese ✔
MSG & Nitrates ✔
Aspartame ✔
Nuts ✔
Onions & Garlic ✔
Yeast ✔

PER SERVING	
Kcals	174
g fat	6
g protein	2
g carbohydrate	28

Middle Eastern Salad

This is a fantastic salad with refreshingly different tastes.

½	cucumber, chopped	½
	salt and pepper	
3-4 tbsp	extra virgin olive oil	3-4 tbsp
1 tbsp	lemon juice	1 tbsp
1	clove garlic, crushed	1
1	tomato, finely chopped	1
½	red pepper, chopped	½
4 tbsp	thinly sliced spring onions	4 tbsp
2 tbsp	finely chopped fresh parsley	2 tbsp
3 tbsp	finely chopped fresh mint	3 tbsp

Put the cucumber in a sieve and sprinkle with a pinch of salt. Leave to drain for 20 minutes, then pat dry.

In large bowl, whisk the olive oil, lemon juice and garlic together with salt and pepper to taste. Stir in the tomato, red pepper, spring onions, parsley and mint. Add the cucumber and toss together. Garnish with mint sprigs and serve with toasted pitta bread or falafel.

Serves 2.

This recipe is FREE of the following triggers (marked ✔)

Caffeine ✔
Chocolate ✔
Citrus fruits
Red wine ✔
Aged cheese ✔
MSG & Nitrates ✔
Aspartame ✔
Nuts ✔
Onions & Garlic
Yeast ✔

PER SERVING	
Kcals	251
g fat	23
g protein	2
g carbohydrate	9

Warm Goats' Cheese Salad with Grilled Vegetables

This tasty salad brings together a wonderful assortment of vegetables. The same amount of English mustard powder can be used instead of Dijon mustard, if MSG is a trigger.

1	small courgette	1
2	small aubergines	2
1	small red or green pepper, seeds removed	1
1	small fennel bulb, top stems removed	1
100 g	goats' cheese log	4 oz
1	egg	1
2 tbsp	water	2 tbsp
50 g	dry breadcrumbs	2 oz
1	bag organic mixed salad greens	1

Optional Salad Dressing

100 ml	raspberry vinegar	4 fl oz
1 tbsp	Dijon mustard	1 tbsp
1 tbsp	herbs (basil, thyme, oregano, etc.)	1 tbsp
175 ml	extra virgin olive oil	6 fl oz
	salt and pepper	

Trim the ends off the courgette and aubergines then cut diagonally lengthways into even-sized pieces.

Cut the pepper lengthways into 2.5 cm/1 inch wide strips.

Cut the fennel bulb into quarters, then cut each quarter in half. Blanch the fennel pieces in boiling salted water for approximately 5 minutes. Set aside.

Cut the goats' cheese into even-sized pieces (see Pointer, next page).

Break the egg into a bowl, and whisk in the water.

Dip the pieces of goats' cheese into the egg wash then press into the breadcrumbs to coat thoroughly all over. Set aside.

For the Salad Dressing, mix the vinegar, mustard and herbs then gradually whisk in the oil. Season with salt and pepper to taste.

This recipe is FREE of the following triggers (marked ✔)

Caffeine ✔
Chocolate ✔
Citrus fruits ✔
Red wine ✔
Aged cheese ✔
MSG & Nitrates
Aspartame ✔
Nuts ✔
Onions & Garlic ✔
Yeast

PER SERVING

Kcals	184
g fat	8
g protein	10
g carbohydrate	18

To assemble the salad, toss the vegetables with a little oil and season with salt and pepper. Fry vegetables over high heat or cook under the grill, turning them over when they are slightly charred, after about 2 minutes.

Meanwhile, pour the dressing over the salad greens and toss to coat thoroughly.

Place equal amounts of salad onto individual plates and arrange the vegetables around the salad. Warm the goats' cheese under the grill for about 1 minute then arrange on top of salad.

Serves 2-4.

Make Ahead: The dressing can be made earlier in the day. It will keep for 1 week if stored in an airtight container in the fridge.

Kitchen Pointer: Try cutting goats' cheese with dental floss – it'll slice it nice and cleanly.

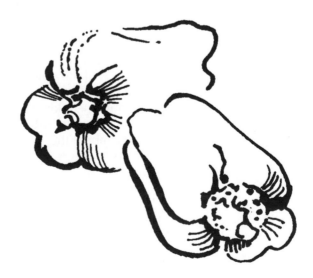

Toasted Creamy Goats' Cheese with Onion Confit

Toasted on aubergine with onion confit, the creamy goats' cheese has a marvellous flavour.

150 ml	olive oil	¼ pint
2	onions, finely sliced	2
3	cloves garlic, finely chopped	3
1	bay leaf	1
4 tbsp	dry white wine (optional)	4 tbsp
2 tbsp	white wine vinegar	2 tbsp
	salt and pepper	
4 tbsp	vegetable oil	4 tbsp
1 tbsp	balsamic vinegar	1 tbsp
2	sprigs fresh rosemary, leaves only, chopped	2
2	sprigs fresh thyme, leaves only, chopped	2
1	aubergine, sliced into rounds	1
350 g	goats' cheese log, cut into 6 rounds	12 oz
1	bag mixed salad greens	1
4 tbsp	vinaigrette dressing	4 tbsp

Heat the olive oil in a frying pan over moderately high heat. Add the onions, half the garlic and bay leaf and cook until onions are transparent. Add the white wine and vinegar. Continue cooking until the confit is reduced by half. Add salt and pepper to taste.

Combine the vegetable oil, remaining garlic, balsamic vinegar, rosemary, thyme, and salt and pepper to taste in a small bowl. Brush this mixture onto the aubergine slices and set aside for 10 minutes. Grill the aubergine slices, turning when slightly charred, for about 2 minutes on each side.

Spread the onion confit over each aubergine slice then top with a slice of goats' cheese. Arrange the aubergine slices on a baking sheet and grill until lightly golden.

Toss the salad greens in vinaigrette then pile onto individual plates and top with the aubergine slices.
Serves 6.

Make Ahead: The onion confit can be prepared a day in advance, or earlier in the day.

PER SERVING	
Kcals	441
g fat	41
g protein	12
g carbohydrate	6

Grilled Portobello Mushrooms with Goats' Cheese and Rocket

The fresh herbs add a wonderful bouquet of flavours to this salad.

4	medium Portobello (field) mushrooms	4
2 tbsp	extra virgin olive oil	2 tbsp
1 tbsp	balsamic vinegar	1 tbsp
½ tsp	chopped garlic	½ tsp
pinch	salt	pinch
1 tsp	each chopped fresh rosemary, thyme and chives	1 tsp
1	bag (100 g) rocket	1
50 g	goats' cheese, crumbled	2 oz
pinch	cracked black pepper	pinch
4	leaves fresh basil, shredded	4

Brush mushrooms with half the olive oil and grill under moderately high heat, turning frequently. When mushrooms begin to release their water, remove them from the heat and set aside. Keep warm.

Whisk together the remaining olive oil, vinegar, garlic, salt and herbs, except the basil.

To Serve
Arrange the rocket leaves on two plates. Toss the warm mushrooms in vinaigrette and place on top of the rocket. Crumble the goats' cheese on top and garnish salad with black pepper and basil leaves.
Serves 2.

Kitchen Pointer: Instead of grilling the mushrooms, you can fry them in a pan over medium heat. To save time, the vinaigrette ingredients can be added straight into the pan when the mushrooms are cooked.

This recipe is FREE of the following triggers (marked ✔)

Caffeine ✓
Chocolate ✓
Citrus fruits ✓
Red wine ✓
Aged cheese ✓
MSG & Nitrates ✓
Aspartame ✓
Nuts ✓
Onions & Garlic
Yeast ✓

PER SERVING	
Kcals	255
g fat	19
g protein	6
g carbohydrate	15

Black-Eyed Bean Salad with Peppers

This unique salad has great flavour, texture, and looks good too.

Vinaigrette

100ml	water	4 fl oz
100 g	raisins, chopped	4 oz
100 ml	fresh lime juice	4 fl oz
6 tbsp	extra virgin olive oil	6 tbsp
2 tbsp	dried oregano	2 tbsp
4 tsp	honey	4 tsp
4 tsp	each ground cumin and coriander	4 tsp
	salt and pepper	

Salad

2	540 ml/19 oz cans black-eyed beans, drained and rinsed	2
100 g	each chopped red pepper, yellow pepper, green pepper, red onion and fresh parsley	4 oz

For the vinaigrette, put the water and raisins into a heavy-based saucepan, and boil for about 2 minutes. Remove from the heat, cover and leave for about 1 hour to soften.

Transfer the raisin mixture to a food processor. Add the lime juice, olive oil, oregano, honey, cumin, and coriander and process until smooth. Season to taste with salt and pepper.

For the salad, toss the beans, peppers, onion and parsley together in a large bowl. Add enough dressing to coat. Season to taste.

Serves 6-8.

Make Ahead: The salad can be made 6 hours ahead and the vinaigrette a day ahead. Before serving, bring to room temperature.

Variation: Substitute different types of beans (cannellini, red) or a combination for even more interest.

PER SERVING (WHEN SERVING 8)	
Kcals	308
g fat	12
g protein	10
g carbohydrate	40

Curried Chicken and Rice Salad with Almonds

This flavourful dish is perfect served cold as a salad, but it can also be served hot as a main course. Worcestershire sauce sometimes contains MSG, so you should be aware of this potential trigger.

<table>
<tr><td>350 g</td><td>basmati rice</td><td>12 oz</td></tr>
<tr><td>350 g</td><td>cooked chicken
(skinless, boneless breasts)</td><td>12 oz</td></tr>
<tr><td>2 tbsp</td><td>olive oil</td><td>2 tbsp</td></tr>
<tr><td>2 tbsp</td><td>plain low-fat yogurt</td><td>2 tbsp</td></tr>
<tr><td>1 tbsp</td><td>curry powder</td><td>1 tbsp</td></tr>
<tr><td>1 tbsp</td><td>light soy sauce (naturally brewed
or Homemade, see p. 125)</td><td>1 tbsp</td></tr>
<tr><td>2 tsp</td><td>wine vinegar</td><td>2 tsp</td></tr>
<tr><td>1 tsp</td><td>celery seeds</td><td>1 tsp</td></tr>
<tr><td>1 tsp</td><td>honey</td><td>1 tsp</td></tr>
<tr><td>1 tsp</td><td>Worcestershire sauce</td><td>1 tsp</td></tr>
<tr><td>½ tsp</td><td>pepper</td><td>½ tsp</td></tr>
<tr><td>350 g</td><td>diced red, yellow or orange pepper</td><td>12 oz</td></tr>
<tr><td>150 g</td><td>slivered almonds</td><td>5 oz</td></tr>
<tr><td>100 g</td><td>diced celery</td><td>4 oz</td></tr>
<tr><td>50 g</td><td>chopped spring onions</td><td>2 oz</td></tr>
<tr><td></td><td>salt and pepper</td><td></td></tr>
</table>

Cook the basmati rice according to packet instructions. Set aside. Dice the chicken and put into a saucepan with the olive oil, yogurt, curry powder, soy sauce, wine vinegar, celery seeds, honey, Worcestershire sauce and pepper. Heat until hot.

Add the rice and remaining ingredients (peppers, almonds, celery and spring onions), cover and simmer for 5 minutes or until vegetables are tender. Season with salt and pepper to taste.

Serves 4.

Variation: If serving the next day as a cold salad, add 1 tbsp plain low-fat yogurt to moisten and 50 g/2 oz shredded carrot. Mix well. Omit spring onions if they are a trigger.

This recipe is FREE of the following triggers (marked ✔)

Caffeine ✔
Chocolate ✔
Citrus fruits ✔
Red wine ✔
Aged cheese ✔
MSG & Nitrates
Aspartame ✔
Nuts
Onions & Garlic
Yeast ✔

PER SERVING

Kcals	722
g fat	26
g protein	25
g carbohydrate	97

Warm Spinach Salad with Prawns

A beautiful and elegant salad bursting with nutrition and flavour.

1	bag (200 g) fresh spinach	1
2 tbsp	olive oil	2 tbsp
8	raw tiger prawns	8
1	red pepper, cut in julienne strips	1
2	tomatoes, seeded and cut in julienne strips	2
4 tbsp	vinegar	4 tbsp
	salt and pepper	

Trim and wash spinach. Pat dry.

Heat the olive oil in a frying pan over moderately high heat. Add the prawns and cook until they turn pink and are firm.

Add the red pepper and tomatoes and cook for 1 minute longer.

Add the spinach and vinegar. Remove from the heat and gently toss. Season with salt and pepper to taste.

Transfer to individual salad plates and serve.

Serves 2.

PER SERVING	
Kcals	217
g fat	14
g protein	11
g carbohydrate	14

Meatless Main Courses

Roasted Wild Mushroom Veggie Burgers

Pasta Salad with Red Peppers and Artichokes

Chinese Noodle Salad with Roasted Aubergine

Vegetable and Cheese Lasagne

Grilled Portobello Mushrooms with Asparagus and Herbed Polenta

Stir-Fried Fresh Vegetables and Tofu

Roasted Wild Mushroom Veggie Burgers

Made with mushrooms and tofu these are a delicious and nutritious vegetarian alternative to beefburgers.

2 tbsp	olive oil	2 tbsp
1	medium onion, chopped	1
pinch	salt	pinch
25 g	dried shiitake mushrooms, soaked in hot water until soft, and drained	1 oz
225 g	wild, button or Portobello mushrooms, (or a mixture), chopped	8 oz
450 g	extra-firm tofu, mashed	1 lb
75 g	quick-cooking oats	3 oz
40 g	toasted wheatgerm	1½ oz
40 g	dry breadcrumbs	1½ oz
2 tbsp	Worcestershire sauce	2 tbsp

Heat the olive oil in a large non-stick frying pan and fry the onion and salt for about 5 minutes.

Remove stalks from shiitake mushrooms. Tip all the mushrooms into a blender or food processor and process until finely chopped.

Add mushroom mixture to the onions and cook for about 10 minutes, stirring occasionally.

Remove mixture from heat and mix with mashed tofu. Add remaining ingredients and mix well. Divide into eight, and with wet hands, shape into burgers.

Place on a greased baking sheet and bake at 190°C/375°F/ Gas Mark 5 for 25 minutes, turning once after 15 minutes.
Serves 8.

This recipe is FREE of the following triggers (marked ✔)

Caffeine ✔
Chocolate ✔
Citrus fruits ✔
Red wine ✔
Aged cheese ✔
MSG & Nitrates
Aspartame ✔
Nuts ✔
Onions & Garlic
Yeast

PER SERVING

Kcals	205
g fat	9
g protein	13
g carbohydrate	18

Pasta Salad with Red Peppers and Artichokes

This colourful and tasty main-course salad is ideal for a cold vegetarian lunch or a light supper.

450 g	fusilli or penne	1 lb
2	medium tomatoes, chopped	2
2	medium red or yellow peppers, chopped	2
100 g	black olives (optional)	4 oz
175 g	marinated artichokes, drained and chopped	6 oz
50 g	grated Parmesan cheese	2 oz
6 tbsp	olive oil	6 tbsp
1 tbsp	red wine vinegar (or cider vinegar)	1 tbsp
2 tsp	Dijon mustard (or 1 tsp of English mustard powder if MSG is a trigger)	2 tsp
2-3	cloves garlic, peeled and chopped	2-3
	salt and pepper	

Bring a large pan of salted water to the boil. Add the pasta and cook until just tender. Drain and tip into a large mixing bowl.

Add the tomatoes, peppers, olives (if using), artichokes and Parmesan cheese to the pasta and toss together.

For the dressing, whisk the olive oil, vinegar, mustard and garlic together in a small bowl.

Toss the pasta with the dressing. Season with salt and pepper to taste and serve.

Serves 4-6.

PER SERVING	
Kcals	463
g fat	15
g protein	13
g carbohydrate	69

Chinese Noodle Salad with Roasted Aubergine

Here's an elegant dish that combines exciting flavours and textures. Look out for mung beans in Asian supermarkets.

This recipe is FREE of the following triggers (marked ✔)
Caffeine ✔
Chocolate ✔
Citrus fruits ✔
Red wine ✔
Aged cheese ✔
MSG & Nitrates ✔
Aspartame ✔
Nuts ✔
Onions & Garlic
Yeast ✔

Marinade and Noodles

100 ml	dark sesame oil	4 fl oz
100 ml	soy sauce, naturally brewed or Homemade (see p. 125)	4 fl oz
3-4 tbsp	sugar	3-4 tbsp
3 tbsp	balsamic vinegar	3 tbsp
3 tbsp	coriander, chopped	3 tbsp
8-10	spring onions, thinly sliced	8-10
1 tbsp	red pepper oil	1 tbsp
2 tsp	salt	2 tsp
1	425 g/15 oz packet Chinese egg noddles (thinnest available) or linguine	1

Aubergine and Vegetable Garnishes

450 g	small, firm aubergines	1 lb
1 tbsp	grated fresh ginger	1 tbsp
1	clove garlic, chopped	1
1 tsp	salt	1 tsp
100 g	mange tout	4 oz
225 g	bean sprouts	8 oz
3 tbsp	sesame seeds (optional)	3 tbsp
1	medium carrot, peeled, cut into julienne strips	1
	fresh coriander to garnish	

Marinade and Noodles
Combine all the ingredients in a large bowl (except the noodles).
   Stir marinade mixture until sugar dissolves.
   Bring a large pan of unsalted water to boil. Gently pull the noodle strands apart then add them to boiling water. Cook the noodles for about 3 minutes or until just tender.

PER SERVING	
Kcals	577
g fat	25
g protein	16
g carbohydrate	72

and tip into a mixing bowl. Stir the marinade then pour half of it over the noodles and toss. Set the remaining marinade aside.

Aubergine and Vegetable Garnishes
Preheat the oven to 200°C/400°F/Gas Mark 6. Pierce the aubergines then put into a baking dish and bake for 20 minutes, depending on size, or until soft, turning once. Leave to cool, cut in half and peel off the skin. Cut the flesh into 5 mm/¼ inch strips.

Add the ginger and garlic to the reserved marinade. Add the aubergine strips to the marinade, turning to coat. Set aside.

Bring a large pan of salted water to the boil. Blanch the mange tout for 1 minute, remove from the pan with a slotted spoon, then rinse in cold water. Cut off strings and cut into strips. Blanch bean sprouts and rinse in the same way. Tip both onto kitchen paper to drain.

Toast the sesame seeds until lightly coloured and fragrant. Toss the noodles with aubergine strips and half of the sesame seeds.

Pile the noodles onto a platter, top with carrot, mange tout and bean sprouts and garnish with remaining sesame seeds and coriander.

Serves 4-6.

Variations: Substitute sesame seeds with roasted peanuts or cashews. Blanched asparagus tips can be used instead of aubergines, and long red or white radishes, thinly sliced and slivered, can also be part of the garnish.

Vegetable and Cheese Lasagne

A tasty dish that's easy when you use ready-made marinara sauce. If MSG or onion is a trigger, make sure you check the label.

250 ml	bought marinara sauce	9 fl oz
225 g	coarsely chopped plum tomatoes	8 oz
1	medium courgette, thinly sliced	1
3 tbsp	chopped fresh basil (or 1 tbsp dried)	3 tbsp
250 g	ricotta cheese	9 oz
175 g	grated Parmesan cheese, plus extra for serving	6 oz
	salt and pepper	
6	sheets of lasagne	6

Simmer marinara sauce, tomatoes, courgette and basil in a saucepan for about 8 minutes or until courgette is tender, stirring occasionally.

Mix the ricotta and Parmesan, then season with salt and pepper to taste.

Cook the lasagne in a large pan of boiling salted water until just tender. Drain.

Place 2 sheets of lasagne in a large greased square glass baking dish. Spread with a quarter of the cheese mixture, then a quarter of the sauce. Repeat, finishing with a final layer of lasagne, vegetable sauce and the rest of the cheese mixture.

Bake at 190°C/375°F/Gas Mark 5, uncovered, for about 15 minutes or until hot and bubbling. Serve with extra Parmesan if you like.

Serves 2-4.

Variation: You can make this with whatever vegetables you have on hand; for example, mushrooms, spinach and onions could easily be substituted.

PER SERVING	
Kcals	529
g fat	25
g protein	33
g carbohydrate	43

Grilled Portobello Mushrooms with Asparagus and Herbed Polenta

In this hearty dish, the polenta is herbed and eaten soft.

6	medium Portobello or field mushrooms	6
5 tsp	extra virgin olive oil	5 tsp
1	bunch asparagus, washed and peeled	1
2 litres	salted water	3½ pints
450 g	instant polenta	1 lb
25 g	unsalted butter	1 oz
1 tbsp	each fresh rosemary, thyme, and parsley, chopped	1 tbsp
	salt and freshly ground pepper	

Clean the mushrooms and brush with 3 teaspoons of olive oil. Season with salt and pepper to taste.

Bring a deep pan of boiling salted water to the boil. Drop in the asparagus and simmer for 2-3 minutes. Remove asparagus with a slotted spoon and refresh by plunging into a bowl filled with iced cold water. Drain on kitchen paper then brush with 1 teaspoon olive oil.

Arrange the asparagus and mushrooms in a grill pan and grill under medium heat or until just tender. Watch carefully so they don't burn.

Bring a large saucepan of salted water (check the packet of polenta for how much) to the boil then add the remaining 1 teaspoon of olive oil and the polenta. Cook for 6 minutes over medium heat, stirring, or according to packet instructions.

Remove polenta from heat and stir in butter and herbs until smooth.

To serve, spoon polenta onto platter and arrange asparagus and mushrooms over the top. Season with freshly ground pepper.

Serves 6.

Make Ahead: The polenta can be prepared earlier and warmed just prior to serving.

PER SERVING	
Kcals	372
g fat	8
g protein	8
g carbohydrate	67

Stir-Fried Fresh Vegetables and Tofu

This stir-fry can be made with or without the tofu. Either way, the simple sauce adds an excellent flavour. Serve the stir-fry with rice for a complete meal.

6 tbsp	olive oil	6 tbsp
225 g	firm tofu, well drained, cut into 1 cm/½ inch cubes	8 oz
2 tbsp	grated fresh ginger	2 tbsp
3	cloves garlic, crushed	3
300 g	fresh shiitake (or button) mushrooms, stalks trimmed, caps sliced	11 oz
175 g	broccoli florets	6 oz
2	red peppers, cut into strips	2
2	bunches spring onions, cut into 2.5 cm/1 inch pieces	2
150 ml	dry white wine	¼ pint
4 tbsp	soy sauce, naturally brewed or Homemade (see p. 125)	4 tbsp
1 tbsp	sesame oil	1 tbsp
	salt and pepper	

Heat 3 tablespoons of the olive oil in a large non-stick frying pan or wok over high heat. Add the tofu and cook, stirring gently, for about 4 minutes or until it starts to brown around the edges. Transfer to a bowl.

Add the remaining oil, ginger, and garlic to the frying pan and stir for about 1 minute. Add the mushrooms and stir-fry for about 5 minutes or until tender around edges. Add the broccoli, red peppers and spring onions and stir-fry for about 3 minutes or until just tender. Add the tofu, white wine, soy sauce and sesame oil and simmer for about 1 minute or until heated through.

Taste and adjust the seasoning before serving.
Serves 4.

PER SERVING	
Kcals	490
g fat	30
g protein	18
g carbohydrate	32

Meat and Poultry

Homestyle Quick Chicken Curry

Simple Chicken Kiev

Curried Chicken with Peaches and Coconut

Japanese-Glazed Chicken

Pasta with Chicken, Asparagus, and Sweet Red Pepper

Chicken Kebabs with Homemade Barbecue Sauce

Poached Chicken with Wild Rice and Baby Vegetables

Roast Duck with Spiced Honey

Filo-Wrapped Chicken with Mushrooms and Spinach in Citron Vodka Sauce

Swedish Meatballs

Sweet and Sour Pork Chops

Pork Fillet with Fresh Tomato Sauce

Quick Lamb Patties

Honey-Roasted Lamb Fillet with Green Asparagus and Plantain Mash

Homestyle Quick Chicken Curry

This is comfort food at its tastiest and easiest. More vegetables can be added with the onion such as carrot, celery and cauliflower. Also cooked lentils will make the meal more substantial. Omit the meat altogether and substitute any cooked beans for a vegetarian version.

1	onion, chopped	1
1-2	dessert apples, sliced	1-2
1-2 tbsp	oil	1-2 tbsp
	curry powder or paste	
250 ml	water or stock	½ pt
25 g	raisins	1 oz
250 g	leftover cooked chicken	8 oz

Fry onion and apple in oil for about 5 minutes. Add curry powder or paste, 1 tsp to 1 tbsp, depending on taste.

Stir then add up to 250 ml/½ pint water or stock. Stir well, add raisins and simmer for 10-15 minutes.

Add pieces of chicken about 5 minutes from the end to heat through.
Serves 4.

Serving suggestion: Serve on a bed of cooked brown rice, and accompany with dessicated coconut.

This recipe is FREE of the following triggers (marked ✔)

Caffeine ✔
Chocolate ✔
Citrus fruits ✔
Red wine ✔
Aged cheese ✔
MSG & Nitrates
Aspartame ✔
Nuts ✔
Onions & Garlic
Yeast ✔

PER SERVING	
Kcals	225
g fat	12
g protein	16
g carbohydrate	15

Simple Chicken Kiev

This recipe turns an often complicated classic into a tasty and easy-to-prepare modern-day delight. Serve it with rice.

4	boneless, skinless chicken breasts	4
	salt and pepper	
4 tsp	butter	4 tsp
4 tsp	chopped chives	4 tsp
2	cloves garlic, crushed	2
½ tsp	tarragon	½ tsp
2	eggs	2
2 tsp	water	2 tsp
3 tbsp	plain flour	3 tbsp
50 g	dry breadcrumbs	2 oz

Cover each chicken breast with clingfilm and beat out with a rolling pin. Season with salt and pepper and top each breast with 1 teaspoon butter, 1 teaspoon chives, a quarter of the garlic and a pinch of tarragon. Fold the chicken to enclose the filling completely and secure with toothpicks.

Beat the eggs and water together. Dip the chicken first in the flour then in the egg mixture, then coat in breadcrumbs. Arrange the chicken seam-side up in a greased baking dish.

Bake at 200°C/400°F/Gas Mark 6, for 20 minutes, turning once, or until the juices run clear when the chicken is pierced with fork.

Serves 4.

PER SERVING	
Kcals	278
g fat	10
g protein	32
g carbohydrate	15

Curried Chicken with Peaches and Coconut

For a simple accompaniment, serve this chicken dish with basmati rice.

25 g	butter	1 oz
1 tbsp	oil	1 tbsp
1.5 kg	chicken pieces	3 lb
2 tbsp	chopped onion (omit onion if a trigger)	2 tbsp
1	small clove garlic, chopped (omit if a trigger)	1
225 g	diced peaches, fresh or canned (drained, if canned)	8 oz
175 ml	chicken stock (see p. 122)	6 fl oz
1½ tsp	curry powder	1½ tsp
½ tsp	cumin	½ tsp
¼ tsp	brown sugar	¼ tsp
	salt and pepper	
	peach slices	
	shredded coconut to garnish	

Melt the butter with the oil in a large frying pan over moderately high heat. Add the chicken pieces and brown slowly all over. Remove from the pan.

Add the onion and garlic to the pan and cook for 5 minutes or until onion is transparent. Add the diced peaches then cook, stirring, for 2 minutes.

Mix the stock, curry powder, cumin and sugar in a bowl. Add to the frying pan and simmer for 5 minutes.

Return the chicken to the pan and season to taste. Cover and simmer until tender, about 25-30 minutes. Remove the chicken from the sauce, arrange on a heated serving platter and keep warm.

Add the peach slices to the sauce and simmer until just until glazed. Pour the sauce over the chicken and garnish with the coconut.

Serves 4-6.

This recipe is FREE of the following triggers (marked ✔)

Caffeine ✔
Chocolate ✔
Citrus fruits ✔
Red wine ✔
Aged cheese ✔
MSG & Nitrates ✔
Aspartame ✔
Nuts ✔
Onions & Garlic
Yeast ✔

PER SERVING (WHEN RECIPE SERVES 6)	
Kcals	397
g fat	25
g protein	33
g carbohydrate	10

Right:
Stir-Fried Fresh Vegetables and Tofu (page 34)

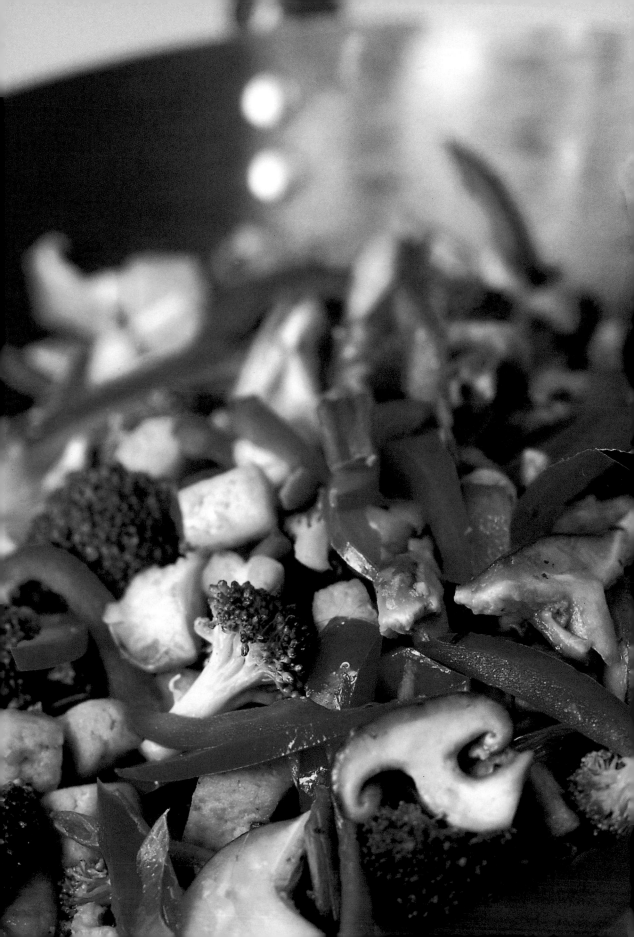

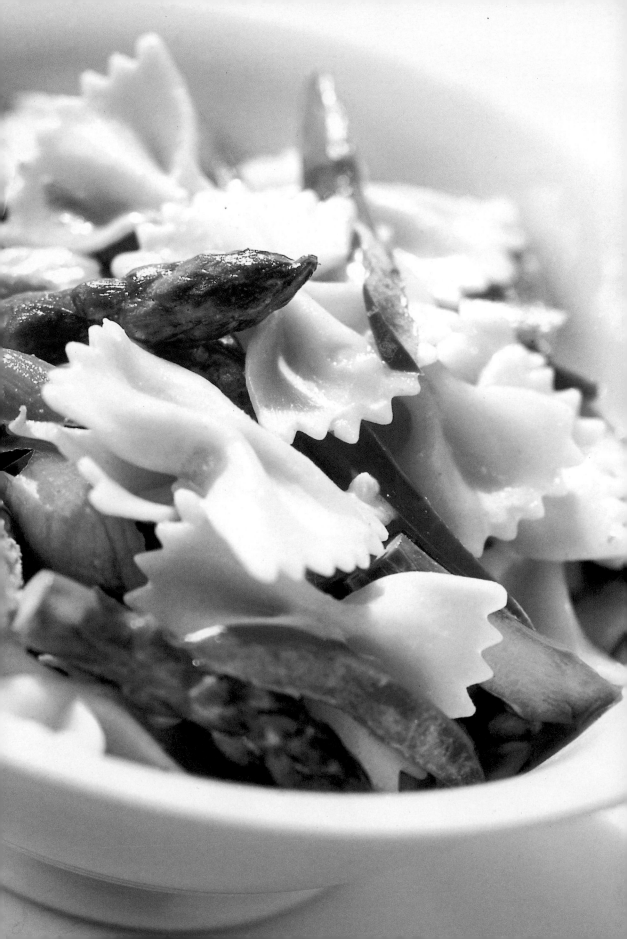

Japanese-Glazed Chicken

This delectable dish is perfect for an Asian-inspired meal. Serve it with rice and mixed vegetables.

8	boneless skinless chicken thighs	8
1	egg	1
100 ml	milk	4 fl oz
50 g	plain flour	2 oz
100 g	sugar	4 oz
125 ml	rice or white wine vinegar	4 fl oz
3 tbsp	water	3 tbsp
3 tbsp	soy sauce, naturally brewed or Homemade (see p. 125)	3 tbsp
1 tsp	salt	1 tsp

Trim the excess fat from the chicken thighs. Beat the egg and milk together. Dip each chicken piece in the egg mixture then coat in flour. Heat a non-stick frying pan until hot then brown the chicken all over for 5 minutes.

Meanwhile, combine remaining ingredients in a bowl. When chicken is browned, arrange in baking dish, large enough to take the chicken in one layer. Pour the soy mixture over the top. Bake at 180°C/350°F/Gas Mark 4 for 1 hour, basting the chicken with the pan juices every 15 minutes.

Serves 4.

This recipe is FREE of the following triggers (marked ✔)

Caffeine ✔
Chocolate ✔
Citrus fruits ✔
Red wine ✔
Aged cheese ✔
MSG & Nitrates ✔
Aspartame ✔
Nuts ✔
Onions & Garlic ✔
Yeast ✔

PER SERVING

Kcals	480
g fat	8
g protein	36
g carbohydrate	66

Left:
Pasta with Chicken, Asparagus and Sweet Red Pepper (page 40)

Pasta with Chicken, Asparagus, and Sweet Red Pepper

The mustard and rosemary give this pasta dish a beautifully mellow flavour.

<table>
<tr><td>450 g</td><td>farfalle (bowtie) pasta</td><td>1 lb</td></tr>
<tr><td>2</td><td>boneless skinless chicken breasts</td><td>2</td></tr>
<tr><td>1</td><td>bunch asparagus</td><td>1</td></tr>
<tr><td>1</td><td>sweet red pepper</td><td>1</td></tr>
<tr><td>3 tbsp</td><td>olive oil</td><td>3 tbsp</td></tr>
<tr><td>2 tbsp</td><td>Dijon mustard (or 1 tbsp English mustard powder if MSG is a trigger)</td><td>2 tbsp</td></tr>
<tr><td>2</td><td>cloves garlic, chopped</td><td>2</td></tr>
<tr><td>1 tbsp</td><td>chopped fresh rosemary</td><td>1 tbsp</td></tr>
<tr><td>150 ml</td><td>dry white wine (optional)</td><td>¼ pint</td></tr>
<tr><td>250 ml</td><td>whipping cream</td><td>9 fl oz</td></tr>
<tr><td></td><td>salt and pepper</td><td></td></tr>
</table>

Bring a large pan of salted water to the boil, add the pasta and cook until tender but still firm. Drain and set aside.

Cut the chicken into bite-sized pieces and set aside.

Wash and cut the asparagus into 2.5 cm/1 inch pieces and set aside.

Cut the red pepper in half, take out the seeds and cut lengthways into thin strips. Set aside.

Heat the oil in a frying pan over moderate heat. Add the chicken and cook for 5 minutes, stirring. Add the asparagus and cook for another 2 minutes. Add the Dijon mustard, garlic, rosemary and red pepper and cook for 1 minute.

Add the white wine (if using), turn up the heat slightly and reduce the liquid by half. Add the cream and reduce until the mixture begins to thicken. Season to taste with salt and pepper.

Add the pasta, stir and heat until the pasta is hot. Serve straight away.

Serves 4-6.

This recipe is FREE of the following triggers (marked ✔)

Caffeine ✔
Chocolate ✔
Citrus fruits ✔
Red wine ✔
Aged cheese ✔
MSG & Nitrates
Aspartame ✔
Nuts ✔
Onions & Garlic
Yeast ✔

PER SERVING

Kcals	269
g fat	17
g protein	11
g carbohydrate	18

Chicken Kebabs with Homemade Barbecue Sauce

The deep and mellow flavour of the barbecue sauce makes it the perfect accompaniment to grilled chicken. Serve these kebabs on a bed of steamed rice. Many brands of mustard and ketchup contain MSG, so watch for these potential triggers.

Barbecue Sauce

6	cloves garlic, crushed	6
1	medium onion, chopped	1
250 ml	tomato ketchup	9 fl oz
3 tbsp	water	3 tbsp
3 tbsp	maple syrup	3 tbsp
3 tbsp	Dijon mustard (or 1 ½ tbsp English mustard powder if MSG is a trigger)	3 tbsp
3 tbsp	balsamic vinegar	3 tbsp
2 tbsp	molasses	2 tbsp
1 tsp	each chopped fresh thyme, rosemary, basil, marjoram and oregano	1 tsp
1 tsp	ground cumin	1 tsp

Kebabs

10	boneless skinless chicken breasts (each breast cut in half lengthwise, and each strip cut into three)	10
1	each red, yellow and green pepper, each cut into 2.5 cm/1 inch squares	1

Barbecue Sauce
Combine all the ingredients in a bowl and set aside.

Kebabs
Marinate the chicken pieces in half of the barbecue sauce for a few hours or overnight. Soak 20 wooden bamboo skewers in water for a few hours or overnight.

Skewer three pieces of chicken and alternating coloured peppers onto the bamboo skewers.

PER SERVING	
Kcals	167
g fat	3
g protein	28
g carbohydrate	7

Make 20 kebabs, allowing two per person.

Preheat the grill to high. Put the kebabs onto the grill rack and cook for 3-5 minutes each side or until the chicken is cooked through. Baste with the remaining barbecue sauce during grilling.

Serve the kebabs on a bed of steamed rice, or with a green salad.

Serves 10.

Make Ahead: The barbecue sauce can be made 2 days in advance, and the kebabs can be prepared a day in advance. Store in the fridge until ready to grill. Great for the barbecue too.

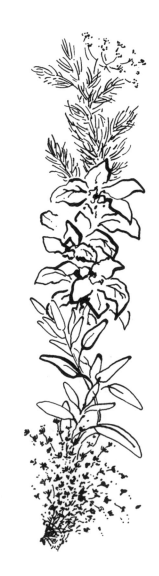

Poached Chicken with Wild Rice and Baby Vegetables

The rich and creamy sauce makes this dish perfect for entertaining.

200 g	mix of wild and long grain rice	7 oz
1 litre	chicken stock (see p. 122)	1¾ pints
4	boneless skinless chicken breasts	4
3	celery stalks, cut into 2.5 cm/1 inch long sticks	3
2	parsnips, peeled, cored and sliced into 5 mm/¼ inch rounds	2
1	carrot, peeled and sliced into 5 mm/¼ inch rounds	1
1	bunch Swiss chard, washed and coarsely chopped	1
250 ml	whipping cream	9 fl oz
	salt and pepper	
1	bunch flat leaf parsley, coarsely chopped	1

Tip the wild and long grain rice mixture into an ovenproof dish that comes with a lid. Pour in enough chicken stock to cover the rice by about 2.5 cm/1 inch. Cover and bake at 230°C/450°F/Gas Mark 8 for about 35 minutes. Remove from the oven and leave to stand for 15 minutes.

Arrange the chicken and vegetables in a large pan, cover with the remaining chicken stock and bring to boil over moderate heat.

Reduce the heat and simmer for about 10 minutes until the chicken is cooked.

Remove the chicken and vegetables from stock, and keep warm and covered. Bring the chicken stock to boil once more then add the cream. Stir frequently until sauce becomes thick enough to coat the spoon. Season with salt and pepper to taste.

To serve, spoon rice onto individual plates, and top with the chicken and vegetables. Garnish with parsley and serve.
Serves 4.

PER SERVING	
Kcals	603
g fat	27
g protein	37
g carbohydrate	53

Roast Duck with Spiced Honey

The succulent flavour of roast duck is combined with the delicious sweetness of honey and spice in this elegant main course.

2	ducks (each 2-2.5 kg/4-5 lb), cut in half lengthways	2
	salt and pepper	
125 ml	honey	4 fl oz
1 tbsp	cumin	1 tbsp
1 tbsp	ground fennel seed	1 tbsp

Preheat the oven to 230°C/450°F/Gas Mark 8.

Place the duck halves, skin side down on a chopping board. Trim any excess fat away with a sharp knife then season generously inside and out with salt and pepper.

Place duck halves, breast side up, on a roasting rack set in shallow baking pan, and roast for 20 minutes. Reduce the heat to 190°C/375°F/Gas Mark 5 and continue roasting for another 20 minutes.

Meanwhile, mix the honey, cumin and fennel seed together in a small bowl to a paste.

Remove the duck halves from oven and baste with the honey-spice mixture. Return to the oven and cook for another 20 minutes or until the skin is very crisp and brown.

Serves 4-6.

Kitchen Pointer: Cooking times may vary depending on the size and weight of the ducks. Check with your butcher and get his advice.

This recipe is FREE of the following triggers (marked ✔)

Caffeine ✓
Chocolate ✓
Citrus fruits ✓
Red wine ✓
Aged cheese ✓
MSG & Nitrates ✓
Aspartame ✓
Nuts ✓
Onions & Garlic ✓
Yeast ✓

PER SERVING
(WHEN RECIPE SERVES 6)

Kcals	902
g fat	70
g protein	48
g carbohydrate	20

Filo-Wrapped Chicken with Mushrooms and Spinach in Citron Vodka Sauce

Want to try something different? This classic recipe combines the delicate flavours of chicken, mushrooms and spinach with the zesty taste of lemon. If lemon juice is a trigger, try using extra amounts of lemon grass.

1	bag (200 g) fresh spinach, trimmed	1
2	boneless skinless chicken breasts, lightly beaten	2
100 g	sliced button mushrooms	4 oz
50 g	butter, melted plus extra for brushing	2 oz
200 g	cooked rice	7 oz
4	sheets filo pastry	4
pinch	salt	pinch
Sauce		
250 ml	whipping cream	9 fl oz
125 ml	chicken stock (see p. 122)	4 fl oz
1 tsp	lemon juice	1 tsp
1 tsp	lemon grass, finely chopped (optional)	1 tsp
2 tbsp	citron vodka (optional)	2 tbsp
	salt	

Rinse the spinach, shake off the excess water and place in saucepan. Cook the spinach, uncovered, until wilted. Drain, squeeze out the excess moisture and chop.

Fry the chicken breasts in a large frying pan until browned on both sides, lifting them now and again to make sure they don't stick. Remove from the pan and leave to cool slightly.

Add the mushrooms and butter to the pan and fry until the mushrooms are softened. Add the rice and chopped spinach to mushrooms. Let cool slightly.

Brush one filo sheet with melted butter. Place second sheet on top and brush lightly with more butter. Repeat with other two filo sheets.

Divide the spinach and rice mixture between the pastry sheets and top each with a chicken breast. Carefully fold

PER SERVING	
Kcals	531
g fat	35
g protein	22
g carbohydrate	32

over the edges of the pastry and press to seal. Put onto a lightly greased baking tray.

Bake at 200°C/400°F/Gas Mark 6 for about 15-20 minutes or until chicken is cooked through and the pastry is golden brown. Meanwhile, bring the sauce ingredients to the boil in a saucepan, then simmer for a few minutes until lightly thickened. Add vodka to the sauce, if using.

Season with salt to taste. If you can't get hold of lemon grass, use basil, thyme, or a mixture of lemon zest and thyme. To serve, pour the sauce onto individual plates and top with a chicken parcel.

Serves 2.

Make Ahead: Follow the recipe and wrap the chicken in the filo earlier in the day. Wrap tightly in clingfilm and keep in the fridge until you want to start cooking.

Swedish Meatballs

This classic dish is a wonderful combination of spiced beef in a creamy sauce. Serve with rice or noodles, a crisp green salad, and crusty bread to mop up the sauce.

100 g	fresh breadcrumbs	4 oz
600 ml	milk	1 pint
900 g	lean minced beef	2 lb
2	eggs, lightly beaten	2
1½ tsp	salt	1½ tsp
¼ tsp	pepper	¼ tsp
1 tsp	nutmeg	1 tsp
100 g	butter	4 oz
40 g	plain flour	1½ oz
750 ml	beef stock (see p. 122)	1¼ pints
350 ml	single cream	12 fl oz

Put the breadcrumbs into a large bowl and pour over just under half the milk. Mix until softened. Add the beef, eggs and seasonings and mix well. Shape into 2.5 cm/1 inch balls. Brown the meatballs all over in butter in a large frying pan. Remove from pan and set aside.

Stir the flour into the fat in the pan. Gradually stir in the stock, the remaining milk and the cream. Simmer over gentle heat for about 3 minutes, stirring constantly.

Add the meatballs to the sauce and simmer for 10-15 minutes or until heated through, stirring occasionally.

Serves 6-8.

PER SERVING (WHEN RECIPE SERVES 6)	
Kcals	564
g fat	40
g protein	31
g carbohydrate	20

Sweet and Sour Pork Chops

This tangy dish is delicious served with potatoes and spinach.

175 ml	water	6 fl oz
100 g	brown sugar	4 oz
100 ml	tomato ketchup	4 fl oz
100 ml	white wine vinegar	4 fl oz
2 tbsp	Worcestershire sauce	2 tbsp
1 tsp	chilli powder	1 tsp
4-6	pork chops	4-6
2	medium onions, sliced	2

Mix the water, sugar, ketchup, vinegar, Worcestershire sauce and chilli powder together in a bowl.

Place the pork chops in a roasting pan and cover with the onions.

Pour over sauce mixture, cover and cook at 150°C/300°F/ Gas Mark 2 for about 1-1½ hours or until the chops are tender.

Serves 4.

This recipe is FREE of the following triggers (marked ✔)

Caffeine ✔
Chocolate ✔
Citrus fruits ✔
Red wine ✔
Aged cheese ✔
MSG & Nitrates
Aspartame ✔
Nuts ✔
Onions & Garlic
Yeast ✔

PER SERVING	
Kcals	329
g fat	9
g protein	22
g carbohydrate	40

Pork Fillet with Fresh Tomato Sauce

These tender pieces of pork cook quickly and are a perfect accompaniment to this savoury tomato-based sauce.

2 tbsp	olive oil	2 tbsp
450 g	pork fillet (tenderloin), cubed	1 lb
1	green pepper, coarsely chopped	1
1	clove garlic, chopped	1
1	celery stalk, coarsely chopped	1
450 g	tomatoes, seeded and chopped	1 lb
½ tsp	each fresh thyme, oregano and basil	½ tsp
	salt and pepper	
450 g	fettuccine	1 lb

Heat the olive oil in a large frying pan over moderately high heat. Add the pork and fry until browned all over. Remove from pan and keep warm.

In same pan, fry the pepper, garlic and celery until tender. Add the tomatoes, thyme, oregano and basil and simmer for 15 minutes longer.

Return the pork to the pan and cook for another 4-6 minutes. Season with salt and pepper to taste.

Meanwhile, cook the fettucine in a large pan of boiling salted water.

Drain the pasta and serve with the pork mixture spooned over the top. Garnish, if you like, with a sprig of thyme or basil.

Serves 4.

This recipe is FREE of the following triggers (marked ✔)

Caffeine ✔
Chocolate ✔
Citrus fruits ✔
Red wine ✔
Aged cheese ✔
MSG & Nitrates ✔
Aspartame ✔
Nuts ✔
Onions & Garlic
Yeast ✔

PER SERVING	
Kcals	680
g fat	12
g protein	44
g carbohydrate	99

Quick Lamb Patties

Served with new potatoes and asparagus, these mint-flavoured patties make a great meal.

300 g	minced lamb	11 oz
1	spring onion, finely chopped	1
1	clove garlic, finely chopped	1
2 tbsp	minced fresh mint	2 tbsp
	salt and pepper	

Preheat the grill. Mix the lamb, spring onion, garlic and mint in a small bowl. Season with salt and pepper and squeeze the mixture between your fingers. Shape the mixture into two 2.5 cm/1 inch patties.

Put the patties on the grill rack in the grill pan and grill for about 4 minutes or until brown. Turn over and grill for about another 4 minutes or until cooked through and browned. **Serves 2.**

This recipe is FREE of the following triggers (marked ✔)

Caffeine ✔
Chocolate ✔
Citrus fruits
Red wine ✔
Aged cheese ✔
MSG & Nitrates ✔
Aspartame ✔
Nuts ✔
Onions & Garlic
Yeast ✔

PER SERVING

Kcals	309
g fat	21
g protein	27
g carbohydrate	3

Honey-Roasted Lamb Fillet with Green Asparagus and Plantain Mash

Delectable pieces of lamb are combined with a honey glaze and mixed with fresh green asparagus and the succulent flavour of roasted plantain.

2 tbsp	honey	2 tbsp
2 tbsp	balsamic vinegar	2 tbsp
4	lamb fillets (tenderloin)	4
2	ripe plantain, skinned and chopped	2
1 tsp	olive oil	1 tsp
	salt and pepper	
4 tbsp	vegetable stock (see p. 121)	4 tbsp
250 ml	whipping cream, reduced by half	9 fl oz
2 tbsp	vegetable oil	2 tbsp
20-25	asparagus spears, trimmed to about 10 cm/4 inch lengths	20-25

Mix the honey and balsamic vinegar together in a small bowl. Coat the lamb with this mixture and leave to marinate for 1-2 hours.

Preheat the oven to 200°C/400°F/Gas Mark 6. Put the plantain, olive oil, salt and pepper into a roasting pan, cover with foil and roast for 10 minutes.

Add the vegetable stock to the plantain (reserve a bit of stock for mashing stage). Continue roasting for 5-7 minutes or until the plantain is very soft. Remove from the oven.

Tip the plantain into a blender and reduce to mash. Add the cream in a steady stream. Add any extra vegetable stock if the mash is too thick. Keep warm.

Remove lamb from the marinade and season well with salt and pepper. Heat the vegetable oil in a non-stick frying pan, add the lamb and brown all over. Remove the lamb from the pan and keep warm. Drain off most of the fat from pan. Add the asparagus and cook for about 3-5 minutes, stirring occasionally, until bright green and tender.

Serve lamb with the asparagus and plantain mash.
Serves 4.

Make Ahead: The plantain mash can be made earlier in the day. Keep covered. Once cooled, put in the fridge until needed. Reheat before serving.

PER SERVING	
Kcals	355
g fat	15
g protein	18
g carbohydrate	37

Fish and Seafood

Fresh Tuna with Maple Mustard Sauce and Coriander Oil

Kedgeree

Herb-Crusted Salmon Fillets

Poached Salmon in Rosé Wine

Grilled Salmon Steaks with Mango Strawberry Coriander Chutney

Salmon Wrapped in Rice Paper in a Yellow Pepper Sauce

Pan-Fried Trout with Cucumber and Prawn Salsa

Baked Halibut with Dill Crust and Red Pepper Sauce

Lemon Sole with Oranges and Honey

Scallops with White Wine and Tarragon Sauce

Grilled Prawns with Two Marinades

Prawn and Carrot Risotto

Portuguese Seafood Risotto

Fresh Tuna with Maple Mustard Sauce and Coriander Oil

Do you want to test your culinary skills? This sophisticated recipe uses raw fish and requires that you build towers!

Coriander Oil

50 g	chopped fresh coriander	2 oz
2 tbsp	chopped fresh parsley	2 tbsp
125 ml	olive oil	4 fl oz

Maple Mustard Sauce

2 tbsp	Dijon mustard, (or half the amount of English mustard powder, if MSG is a trigger)	2 tbsp
1 tbsp	maple syrup	1 tbsp
1 tbsp	fresh lemon juice	1 tbsp
2 tsp	sherry vinegar	2 tsp
4 tbsp	vegetable oil	4 tbsp

Tuna

1	avocado, peeled, stoned, and diced	1
2 tbsp	lemon juice	2 tbsp
	salt and pepper	
1	mango, peeled, stoned, and diced	1
2 tbsp	coriander oil (ingredients above, method follows)	2 tbsp
2	plum tomatoes, seeded and chopped	2
100 g	fresh tuna, thinly diced	4 oz
2 tbsp	finely chopped onions	2 tbsp
1 tsp	each mirin and tamari (optional)	1 tsp
3 tbsp	chopped chives	3 tbsp
1	frisée lettuce	1
4 tsp	salmon roe	4 tsp
2	175 g/6 oz tuna steaks (centre cut)	2

PER SERVING (WHEN RECIPE SERVES 4)	
Kcals	699
g fat	55
g protein	30
g carbohydrate	21

Coriander Oil

Blanch the coriander and parsley in a small pan of boiling water for 30-60 seconds until bright green. Drain, plunge into cold water, and drain again. Dry in salad spinner or on kitchen paper.

Purée the coriander and parsley in a blender until smooth. Add the oil in a steady stream and blend for 3-4 minutes. Pass through a fine sieve or a piece of muslin and set aside.

Maple Mustard Emulsion

Whisk the mustard, maple syrup, lemon juice and sherry vinegar together in a small bowl. Still whisking, gradually drizzle in oil. Set aside.

Tuna

Mix the avocado, lemon juice and salt and pepper to taste in a small bowl.

In another small bowl, stir the mango, 1 tbsp coriander oil and salt and pepper to taste.

In a third bowl, mix the tomatoes with 1 tbsp coriander oil and salt and pepper to taste.

Toss the diced tuna, onions, mirin, tamari (if using), chives, and salt and pepper to taste.

To Assemble

Using a 7.5 cm/3 inch round pastry cutter, build a tower in the centre of each dinner plate by packing a quarter of the avocado mixture into the ring, followed by quarter each of mango, tomato and fish mixtures. Pack lightly and gently remove ring.

Top each tower with equal amounts of frisée and a spoonful of salmon roe.

Arrange the fish steaks around tower then drizzle with the remaining coriander oil and maple mustard sauce.
Serves 2-4.

Kitchen Pointer: Mirin is a fermented rice wine with a trace of alcohol. Tamari is Japanese soy sauce.

Make Ahead: Towers can be made 1 hour or more ahead, covered with clingfilm and chilled. You can use salmon or salmon trout instead of the tuna.

Kedgeree

An old fashioned fish and rice dish that used to be served for breakfast. It makes a good light family lunch or supper dish.

250 g	long grain rice	8 oz
1 tbsp	oil	1 tbsp
600 ml	boiling water or fish stock	1 pint
1	stalk celery	1
50 g	butter	2 oz
600 ml	milk	1 pint
2	fillets cooked, smoked fish of your choice	2
1-2	hard-boiled eggs	1-2
	salt and pepper	
	chopped parsley, optional	

Turn the rice in oil over a gentle heat. Add boiling water or stock and simmer slowly until all the water is absorbed and the rice cooked.

Flake the butter into the rice, and stir it in. Flake in the fish, and chopped hard-boiled egg.

Test and season to taste, adding chopped parsley if liked. **Serves 4.**

Variation: A pinch of turmeric in the rice cooking water will make the rice yellow, which is attractive. A cheaper white fish can be used, but most often it is served with smoked haddock. For something special you could go to town with smoked salmon and prawns. Try adding a little grated lemon rind, and offer slices of lemon to squeeze the juice over.

PER SERVING	
Kcals	409
g fat	17
g protein	17
g carbohydrate	51

Herb-Crusted Salmon Fillets

The piquant-flavoured crust of capers, horseradish and fresh herbs pairs wonderfully with the mellow richness of roasted salmon. Horseradish is in the onion family, though, so watch for this potential trigger.

2 tbsp	parsley, leaves only	2 tbsp
2 tbsp	chopped chives	2 tbsp
1 tbsp	capers	1 tbsp
1 tbsp	fresh tarragon, leaves only	1 tbsp
2 tsp	Dijon mustard (or 1 tsp English mustard powder, if MSG is a trigger)	2 tsp
2 tsp	Worcestershire sauce (optional)	2 tsp
100 g	fresh breadcrumbs from white loaf	4 oz
2 tbsp	fresh horseradish, peeled and grated	2 tbsp
	salt and pepper	
4	salmon fillets (175 g/6 oz each)	4

Put the parsley, chives, capers, tarragon, mustard and Worcestershire sauce into a food processor and process for about 2 minutes or until smooth.

Transfer the purée to a mixing bowl. Add the breadcrumbs, horseradish and salt and pepper to taste.

Mix until well combined – the mixture should be moist, but hold together when you squeeze it. If it is too wet, add more breadcrumbs. If too dry, add water.

Preheat the oven to 200°C/400°F/Gas Mark 6. Put the salmon on a lightly oiled baking sheet. Divide the herb topping between the fish, packing it down firmly. Bake for 15 minutes or until the fish flakes easily when tested with fork (less if you prefer salmon slightly rare).

Serves 4.

Make Ahead: The herb breadcrumb mixture can be prepared earlier in the day. If you would like a more generous crust, double the amount.

This recipe is FREE of the following triggers (marked ✔)

Caffeine ✔
Chocolate ✔
Citrus fruits ✔
Red wine ✔
Aged cheese ✔
MSG & Nitrates
Aspartame ✔
Nuts ✔
Onions & Garlic
Yeast

PER SERVING	
Kcals	416
g fat	20
g protein	37
g carbohydrate	22

Poached Salmon in Rosé Wine

Nothing could be more elegant than whole salmon poached in fragrant rosé wine and served with Hollandaise Sauce.

1 litre	water	1¾ pints
2	chopped shallots	2
1	stalk celery with leaves, chopped	1
1	carrot, chopped	1
1	bunch fresh parsley	1
1 tsp	salt	1 tsp
600 ml	rosé wine	1 pint
1	whole salmon (2-2.5 kg/4-5 lb)	1
2	lemons, cut into wedges	2
	Hollandaise Sauce (p. 124)	

Bring the water, shallots, celery, carrot, four sprigs of parsley and salt to the boil in a saucepan over medium-high heat. Reduce the heat then simmer, uncovered, for 20 minutes.

Pour this stock into a fish kettle or large roasting pan. Add the wine.

Wash the fish inside and out. Put on a rack and into pan. The fish should be at least half covered by liquid – if not, just add more water or wine to the pan.

Bring the liquid to just under boiling point so that water appears to shiver rather than bubble. (If you cook fish faster than this, it will tend to fall apart.)

Poach, covered, for 35 minutes or just until fish flakes easily when tested with fork.

Carefully lift the rack with the fish on it out of the pan. Remove any bits of vegetables. Arrange the fish on a platter and garnish with lemon wedges and remaining parsley. Serve with Hollandaise Sauce.

Serves 10.

Variation: You can substitute salmon with red snapper.

PER SERVING (WITH 2 TBSP HOLLANDAISE SAUCE)	
Kcals	330
g fat	22
g protein	33
g carbohydrate	trace

Grilled Salmon Steaks with Mango Strawberry Coriander Chutney

The tanginess of strawberries and the sweetness of mango are the perfect combination for grilled salmon. Serve this dish with wild rice and ratatouille.

<table>
<tr><td>2</td><td>nearly ripe mangoes</td><td>2</td></tr>
<tr><td>350 g</td><td>strawberries</td><td>12 oz</td></tr>
<tr><td>1</td><td>sweet red pepper, seeds removed</td><td>1</td></tr>
<tr><td>1</td><td>bunch coriander</td><td>1</td></tr>
<tr><td>150 ml</td><td>water or white wine</td><td>¼ pint</td></tr>
<tr><td>2 tbsp</td><td>honey</td><td>2 tbsp</td></tr>
<tr><td>2 tbsp</td><td>curry powder</td><td>2 tbsp</td></tr>
<tr><td>1 tbsp</td><td>cinnamon</td><td>1 tbsp</td></tr>
<tr><td>2</td><td>salmon steaks (175 g/6 oz each)</td><td>2</td></tr>
<tr><td></td><td>olive or vegetable oil</td><td></td></tr>
<tr><td></td><td>salt and pepper</td><td></td></tr>
</table>

Cut the mangoes down either side of the stone and remove flesh from the skin in cubes. Hull the strawberries, cut into quarters, and cut the red pepper into cubes. Coarsely chop the coriander.

Put the red pepper in small saucepan and cook for one minute. Add mango, water or wine, honey, curry powder and cinnamon.

Reduce the heat to low and simmer for about 10 minutes or until the mixture is syrupy.

Add the strawberries and coriander and simmer for 2 minutes more.

Rub salmon steaks with oil, season with salt and pepper to taste, and fry or grill, for 3 minutes on either side. Arrange the salmon on individual plates and serve with the mango chutney.

Serves 2.

Make ahead: The chutney can be prepared earlier in the day. Store it in the fridge and bring it to room temperature just before serving.

This recipe is FREE of the following triggers (marked ✔)

Caffeine ✔
Chocolate ✔
Citrus fruits ✔
Red wine ✔
Aged cheese ✔
MSG & Nitrates ✔
Aspartame ✔
Nuts ✔
Onions & Garlic ✔
Yeast ✔

PER SERVING

Kcals	342
g fat	18
g protein	34
g carbohydrate	11

Salmon Wrapped in Rice Paper in a Yellow Pepper Sauce

The fresh taste of ginger and garlic blends beautifully with salmon. Serve this exotic dish with a fresh green salad. The commercially made sauces may contain MSG, so read the labels carefully.

4	pieces rice paper	4
450 g	salmon fillet, cut into 4	1 lb
4	sprigs each basil and coriander	4
Marinade		
2	cloves garlic, finely chopped	2
1 tbsp	chopped coriander	1 tbsp
2 tsp	chopped fresh ginger	2 tsp
2 tsp	tamari sauce	2 tsp
1 tsp	each oyster sauce, mirin (optional), and sesame oil	1 tsp
Sauce		
1 tsp	extra virgin olive oil	1 tsp
1	clove garlic	1
1	large shallot, finely chopped	1
2	large yellow peppers, seeded and chopped	2
350 ml	fish or vegetable stock	12 fl oz
	salt and pepper	

Marinade
Mix all the ingredients together in a bowl.
   Pour the mixture over the salmon fillets and leave to marinate for about 1 hour.

Sauce
Heat the oil in saucepan over medium heat, add the garlic and shallot and fry until softened. Add the peppers and the stock, stirring well.
   Cover and simmer for 20 minutes or until the peppers are tender.
   Leave to cool slightly, then process in a food processor until the mixture is smooth. Season with salt and pepper to taste. Set aside.

This recipe is FREE of the following triggers (marked ✔)

Caffeine ✔
Chocolate ✔
Citrus fruits ✔
Red wine ✔
Aged cheese ✔
MSG & Nitrates
Aspartame ✔
Nuts ✔
Onions & Garlic
Yeast ✔

PER SERVING	
Kcals	319
g fat	15
g protein	27
g carbohydrate	19

To Assemble

Remove the fish from the marinade. Dry gently removing excess ingredients. Season with salt and pepper to taste.

Dip each piece of rice paper in water until workable. Wrap each salmon fillet in rice paper with sprigs of basil and coriander. Steam the fish in a bamboo steamer set above a pan of rapidly boiling water, or in a fish steamer, for 3 to 4 minutes.

Reheat the yellow pepper sauce and spoon onto individual plates. Place salmon on top of sauce.

Serves 4.

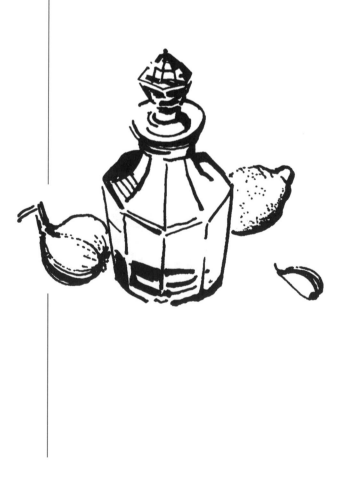

Pan-Fried Trout with Cucumber and Prawn Salsa

The fresh ingredients are what makes this dish so spectacular. Serve it with rice, potatoes or noodles and your favourite vegetable.

4	trout or salmon trout	4
Salsa		
225 g	cooked prawns, shelled	8 oz
1	red onion, diced	1
½	mango, sliced	½
½	sweet red pepper, diced	½
1	cucumber (½ diced, ½ sliced)	1
2 tbsp	rice wine vinegar	2 tbsp
2 tbsp	olive oil	2 tbsp
1 tbsp	chopped fresh dill	1 tbsp
	additional oil for frying trout	
	salt and pepper	

For the salsa, mix the prawns, onion, mango, red pepper, diced cucumber, rice vinegar, olive oil and dill together (keep the sliced cucumber for garnish). Chill in the fridge.

Heat enough olive oil to generously cover the base of a large frying pan. Season the trout with salt and pepper inside and out, and fry for 4-5 minutes on each side.

Transfer the trout to a warm plate and garnish with cucumber slices. Top with salsa and serve hot.

Serves 4.

Make Ahead: Prepare the salsa earlier in the day and chill.

This recipe is FREE of the following triggers (marked ✔)

Caffeine ✔
Chocolate ✔
Citrus fruits ✔
Red wine ✔
Aged cheese ✔
MSG & Nitrates ✔
Aspartame ✔
Nuts ✔
Onions & Garlic
Yeast ✔

PER SERVING	
Kcals	361
g fat	17
g protein	42
g carbohydrate	10

Baked Halibut with Dill Crust and Red Pepper Sauce

Sometimes it is the simplest ingredients that bring out the best in fish. Fresh dill, red pepper, garlic and olive oil help to create a uniquely flavourful dish.

This recipe is FREE of the following triggers (marked ✔)

Caffeine ✔
Chocolate ✔
Citrus fruits ✔
Red wine ✔
Aged cheese ✔
MSG & Nitrates ✔
Aspartame ✔
Nuts ✔
Onions & Garlic
Yeast ✔

Halibut Fillets

225 g	halibut fillets	8 oz
1 tsp	olive oil	1 tsp
2 tsp	chopped fresh dill	2 tsp
	salt and pepper	

Place fish fillets on a large piece of foil, drizzle with olive oil then top with the dill and salt and pepper to taste.

Wrap the fillets tightly in the foil and place on a baking sheet. Bake at 190°C/375°F/Gas Mark 5 for 10-12 minutes or until fish flakes easily when tested with fork.

Serve with Red Pepper Sauce (below).

Red Pepper Sauce

1	red pepper, seeded	1
1	clove garlic, chopped	1
1 tbsp	olive oil	1 tbsp
	salt and pepper	

Cut the pepper into large pieces then toss with the garlic and the oil in a small bowl.

Spread out on a baking sheet, skin side up, and roast in the oven with the fish until soft and charred. Remove the skins.

Process in a food processor until smooth. Pass through sieve and season with salt and pepper to taste.

Serves 2.

PER SERVING	
Kcals	224
g fat	12
g protein	26
g carbohydrate	3

Lemon Sole with Oranges and Honey

In this wonderful recipe, the delicate flavour of lemon sole is paired with the tanginess of oranges and the sublime sweetness of honey.

175g	wild rice	6 oz
25 g	butter	1 oz
4	shallots, finely chopped	4
300 ml	dry white wine	½ pint
300 ml	orange juice	½ pint
2 tsp	grated orange zest	2 tsp
	salt and pepper	
	clear honey	
8	lemon sole fillets	8
2 tbsp	plain flour	2 tbsp
	oil for shallow frying	
2	oranges, peeled and segmented	2
2 tbsp	chopped fresh parsley	2 tbsp

Cook the wild rice in a large pan of boiling salted water for 40-45 minutes or according to packet instructions, until tender.

Melt the butter in a large saucepan, add the shallots, and cook for 3 minutes until softened.

Add the wine, orange juice and orange zest. Bring to the boil and continue boiling until reduced by half. Season with salt and pepper to taste. Add honey to taste. Cover and keep warm.

Coat the sole with flour and season well. Heat the oil in a frying pan, then add the fish in batches. Cook for 3 minutes on each side or until fish is opaque. Keep warm.

Drain the rice and stir in the orange segments. Spoon onto warmed serving dish and place fish on top. Pour the sauce over the fish and garnish with parsley.
Serves 4.

PER SERVING	
Kcals	505
g fat	13
g protein	40
g carbohydrate	57

Scallops with White Wine and Tarragon Sauce

Enjoy tender scallops in a creamy herb and wine sauce – without the cream! Serve with rice or pasta.

450 g	scallops (about 16), shelled	1 lb
25 g	butter	1 oz
100 g	shallots, diced	4 oz
2	carrots, diced	2
2 tbsp	finely chopped sweet red pepper	2 tbsp
1	clove garlic, grated	1
2 tbsp	plain flour	2 tbsp
100 ml	dry white wine	4 fl oz
250 ml	skimmed milk	9 fl oz
2 tbsp	chopped fresh parsley	2 tbsp
1 tbsp	chopped fresh tarragon	1 tbsp
	salt and pepper	
2 tbsp	chopped chives	2 tbsp

Rinse the scallops under cold water and dry with kitchen paper.

Melt half the butter in a large frying pan and cook the scallops for 1 minute on each side. Remove from the pan and set aside.

Melt the rest of the butter, add the shallots, carrots and pepper, and fry for 5 minutes. Stir in the garlic and fry for 1 minute. Stir in the flour and cook for another 1 minute. Pour in the wine, stirring constantly.

Gradually add the milk, stirring constantly, until the sauce comes to the boil. Reduce the heat and simmer, stirring occasionally, for 3 minutes.

Stir in the scallops, parsley and tarragon. Cook for 30 seconds. Season to taste with salt and pepper.
Pour into a serving dish or spoon onto plates and garnish with chopped chives.
Serves 4.

Variation: Substitute fresh dill for tarragon.

This recipe is FREE of the following triggers (marked ✔)

Caffeine ✔
Chocolate ✔
Citrus fruits ✔
Red wine ✔
Aged cheese ✔
MSG & Nitrates ✔
Aspartame ✔
Nuts ✔
Onions & Garlic
Yeast ✔

PER SERVING	
Kcals	215
g fat	7
g protein	23
g carbohydrate	15

Grilled Prawns with Two Marinades

If you enjoy the delicate flavours of orange and sesame, then you'll love the orange-sesame marinade. However, if you're in the mood for something a little more assertive, the zestiness of balsamic vinegar might be just the thing.

20	raw tiger prawns, shelled but with tails intact	20
Orange-Sesame Marinade		
3 tbsp	orange juice	3 tbsp
1 tsp	sesame oil	1 tsp
	pepper	
Balsamic Vinegar and Garlic Marinade		
2 tbsp	olive oil	2 tbsp
1½ tsp	balsamic vinegar	1½ tsp
½ tsp	Worcestershire sauce	½ tsp
1	clove garlic, crushed	1
	cayenne pepper	

Mix the ingredients together for your choice of marinade.

Add the prawns and toss to coat. Marinate for 1 hour at room temperature.

Grill or fry under or over medium heat, turning frequently, for about 5 minutes or until the prawns are bright pink. Be careful not to overcook.

Serves 4.

PER SERVING	
Kcals	45
g fat	1
g protein	7
g carbohydrate	2

Prawn and Carrot Risotto

Here's a risotto recipe that combines the earthiness of Arborio rice with tender morsels of prawn and cooked carrot for a dash of colour.

<table>
<tr><td>3</td><td>carrots, peeled and chopped</td><td>3</td></tr>
<tr><td>2 tbsp</td><td>olive oil</td><td>2 tbsp</td></tr>
<tr><td>3</td><td>shallots, sliced</td><td>3</td></tr>
<tr><td>350 g</td><td>Arborio rice</td><td>12 oz</td></tr>
<tr><td>100 ml</td><td>carrot cooking liquid (see recipe)</td><td>4 fl oz</td></tr>
<tr><td>750 ml</td><td>vegetable stock (see p. 121)</td><td>1¼ pints</td></tr>
<tr><td>2</td><td>carrots, grated</td><td>2</td></tr>
<tr><td>40 g</td><td>unsalted butter</td><td>1½ oz</td></tr>
<tr><td>16</td><td>cooked peeled prawns</td><td>16</td></tr>
<tr><td></td><td>salt and pepper</td><td></td></tr>
<tr><td></td><td>parsley, chopped</td><td></td></tr>
</table>

Cook the chopped carrots in a large pan of boiling salted water for 20 minutes or until tender. Strain carrots and reserve 100 ml/4 fl oz cooking liquid for later. Purée the cooked carrots in a food processor until smooth. Place in bowl and set aside.

Heat the olive oil in a large saucepan over medium-high heat. Add the shallots and cook for about 3 minutes.

Add the rice and cook for another 3 minutes. Add the carrot cooking liquid and simmer, stirring occasionally, until liquid has been absorbed.

Add half of the vegetable stock, stirring occasionally, until liquid has been absorbed.

Stir in the carrot purée, grated carrot and remaining vegetable stock. Simmer, stirring, until liquid is absorbed and the risotto is creamy. Add the butter and prawns. Stir until the butter is incorporated and prawns are heated through. Serve on individual dinner plates or on a large serving platter. Garnish with parsley.

Serves 4.

This recipe is FREE of the following triggers (marked ✔)

Caffeine ✔
Chocolate ✔
Citrus fruits ✔
Red wine ✔
Aged cheese ✔
MSG & Nitrates ✔
Aspartame ✔
Nuts ✔
Onions & Garlic
Yeast ✔

PER SERVING	
Kcals	532
g fat	16
g protein	14
g carbohydrate	83

Portuguese Seafood Risotto

A delectable combination of fresh shellfish and firm white fish, this creamy rice dish is best served with generous slices of fresh crusty bread.

125 ml	olive oil	4 fl oz
1	onion, finely chopped	1
3	cloves garlic, finely chopped	3
18	large mussels, scrubbed and bearded	18
12	raw tiger prawns, shelled	12
6	medium to large clams, scrubbed	6
350 g	salmon fillet	12 oz
350 g	monkfish, cubed	12 oz
2	squid, cleaned and cut into rings	2
225 g	Arborio rice	8 oz
300 ml	white wine (optional)	½ pint
500 ml	fish stock (see p. 123) or water	18 fl oz
pinch	saffron	pinch
	salt and pepper	
75 g	butter	3 oz
1 tbsp	chopped coriander	1 tbsp
1 tbsp	lemon juice	1 tbsp

Heat the olive oil in a large deep casserole over moderately-high heat. Add the onion, garlic and all the shellfish and fish. Cook for 2-3 minutes. Remove and set aside all shellfish and fish. Discard any clams and mussels that do not open.

Add the rice to the casserole, and cook, stirring, for 2 minutes. Do not let the rice brown. Add the wine, if using, and cook over high heat until it has evaporated.

Reduce the heat to moderate. Add the fish stock in small amounts, adding more as liquid is absorbed. Add the saffron, and salt and pepper to taste. Stirring constantly, cook for 12-15 minutes or until the rice is creamy and tender but firm. Add additional liquid, if necessary.

Return the shellfish and fish to the risotto and cook for 3 minutes or until heated through. Gently stir in the butter, coriander and lemon juice. Adjust the seasoning if necessary.
Serves 4-6.

PER SERVING (WHEN RECIPE SERVES 6)	
Kcals	662
g fat	38
g protein	41
g carbohydrate	39

Kitchen Pointer: Clams and mussels should be removed as soon as they unclench their shells, otherwise they will become tough. Some shells will open up sooner than others, and the mussels will open up before the clams. Clam and mussel shells that do not open should be discarded.

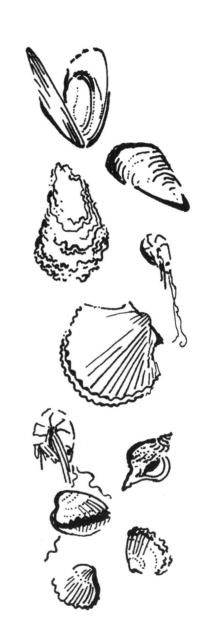

Vegetables and Side Dishes

Stir-Fried Peppers and Bean Sprouts

Roasted Vegetable Medley

Asparagus Spears with Apple, Egg and Poppy Seed Dressing

Charred Courgettes with Herbs, Garlic and Ricotta

Roasted New Potatoes with Herbs

Mushrooms and Rice

Steamed Basmati Rice with Crisp Potatoes, Sumac and Cumin

Herb and Cherry Tabbouleh

Bulgur and Green Bean Salad with Herbed Vinaigrette

Grilled Polenta with Tomato Sauce

Stir-Fried Peppers and Bean Sprouts

This simple and colourful side dish features bright red and green peppers fried with the tanginess of fresh ginger and bean sprouts.

2 tbsp	cooking oil	2 tbsp
1 tsp	grated fresh ginger	1 tsp
½ tsp	salt	½ tsp
1	green pepper, seeded and cut in strips	1
1	red pepper, seeded and cut in strips	1
350 g	bean sprouts	12 oz
4 tbsp	chicken stock (see p. 122)	4 tbsp

Heat the oil in a wok or large frying pan. Add the ginger, salt and peppers and stir-fry for 2 minutes. Add the bean sprouts and stir-fry for 1 minute. Add in the stock, cover and cook for another 2-3 minutes or until the vegetables are tender.

Serves 2.

This recipe is FREE of the following triggers (marked ✔)

Caffeine ✔
Chocolate ✔
Citrus fruits ✔
Red wine ✔
Aged cheese ✔
MSG & Nitrates ✔
Aspartame ✔
Nuts ✔
Onions & Garlic
Yeast ✔

PER SERVING	
Kcals	156
g fat	12
g protein	4
g carbohydrate	8

Right:
Prawn and Carrot Risotto
(page 66)

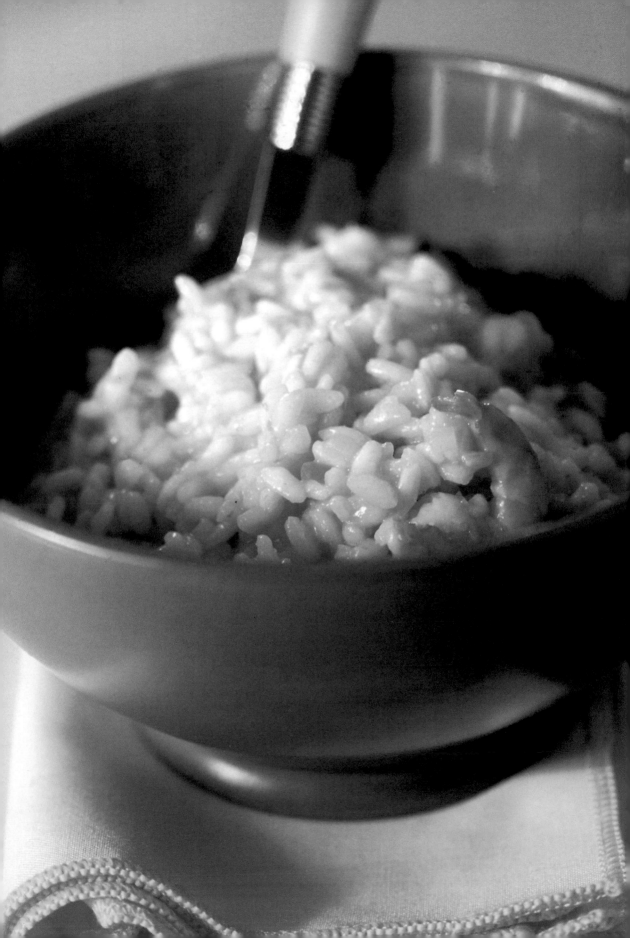

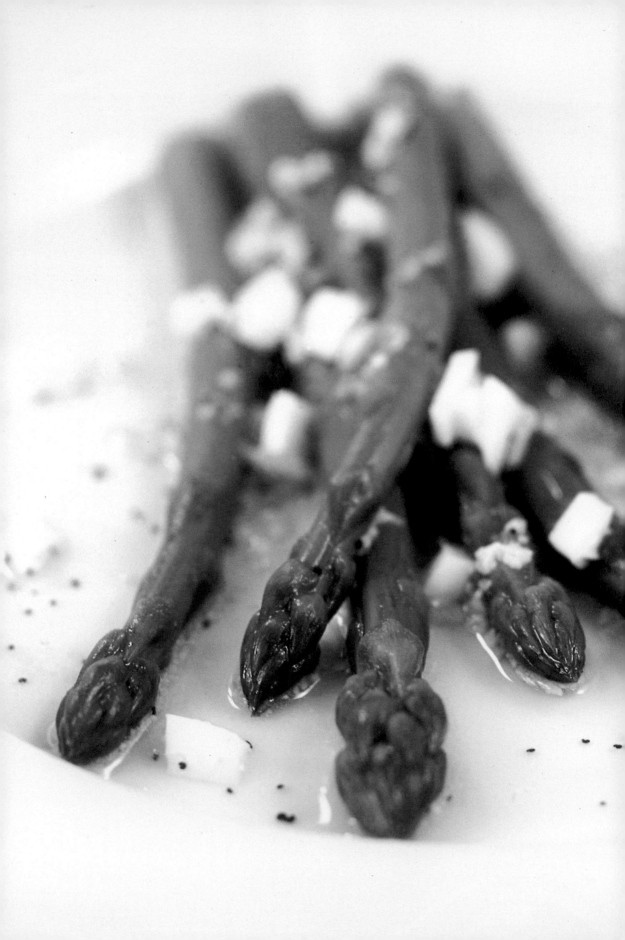

Roasted Vegetable Medley

Roasted in their own juices, these vegetables are tender and very flavourful.

6	small potatoes, peeled if liked, and quartered	6
4	large carrots, peeled if liked, and cut into 7.5 cm/3 inch lengths	4
2	small onions, peeled and quartered	2
2	small courgettes, sliced	2
2 tbsp	olive oil	2 tbsp
1 tsp	thyme	1 tsp
	salt and pepper	

Preheat the oven to 220°C/425°F/Gas Mark 7. Combine the potatoes, carrots, onions and three quarters of the oil in a bowl and toss to mix. In a separate bowl, toss the courgettes with the remaining oil. Put all the vegetables (except the courgettes) in roasting pan. Sprinkle with thyme, and salt and pepper to taste. Roast for about 40 minutes. Add the courgettes and gently turn vegetables. Return pan to the oven and roast for another 15-20 minutes or until vegetables are tender.
Serves 4.

Variations: Parsnips, turnips, fennel, chunks of celeriac or butternut squash also make good vegetables for roasting. Garlic and herbs such as bay leaves can be added for additional flavour.

This recipe is FREE of the following triggers (marked ✔)

Caffeine ✔
Chocolate ✔
Citrus fruits ✔
Red wine ✔
Aged cheese ✔
MSG & Nitrates ✔
Aspartame ✔
Nuts ✔
Onions & Garlic
Yeast ✔

PER SERVING	
Kcals	218
g fat	6
g protein	5
g carbohydrate	36

Left:
Asparagus Spears with Apple, Egg and Poppy Seed Dressing (page 72)

Asparagus Spears with Apple, Egg and Poppy Seed Dressing

This dish is best made in late spring or early summer when asparagus is at its peak. A perfect accompaniment to grilled meats, it also works well as part of antipasto. Make sure you have hard-boiled eggs on hand for this recipe.

24	asparagus spears	24
2	hard-boiled eggs	2
125 ml	apple juice	4 fl oz
2 tbsp	honey	2 tbsp
1 tbsp	poppy seeds	1 tbsp
4 tbsp	cider vinegar	4 tbsp
	salt and pepper	

Snap off the tough ends from the asparagus and peel the stems. Blanch in a large frying pan of boiling water, for about 15-20 seconds or until barely tender. Immediately immerse cooked asparagus in ice water to stop the cooking process. Set aside.

Peel the eggs and separate the yolks from the whites. Grate the yolks. Add the apple juice, honey and poppy seeds. Blend together, using only as much cider vinegar as required to make a pourable sauce and according to taste.

Dice the egg white. Reheat the asparagus in hot water, and drain. Arrange six spears per serving on individual salad plates. Pour the sauce over the asparagus and garnish with diced egg whites.

Serves 4.

This recipe is FREE of the following triggers (marked ✔)

Caffeine ✔
Chocolate ✔
Citrus fruits ✔
Red wine ✔
Aged cheese ✔
MSG & Nitrates ✔
Aspartame ✔
Nuts ✔
Onions & Garlic ✔
Yeast ✔

PER SERVING	
Kcals	131
g fat	3
g protein	6
g carbohydrate	20

Charred Courgettes with Herbs, Garlic and Ricotta

Salting and draining the courgettes prevents excess liquid from watering down this light and tasty side dish.

2	medium green or yellow courgettes	2
	salt	
1 tsp	olive oil	1 tsp
2	fresh thyme sprigs	2
pinch	dried oregano	pinch
1 tbsp	fresh chopped basil (and/or parsley)	1 tbsp
2	cloves garlic, grated	2
100 g	ricotta or goats' cheese	4 oz
1 tsp	dry breadcrumbs	1 tsp
1 tsp	melted butter	1 tsp

Cut the courgettes in half lengthways. Sprinkle with salt and set aside for about 20 minutes. Dry the courgettes with kitchen paper then coat with olive oil.

Grill or fry the courgette halves over or under high heat for about 3 minutes. Toss immediately with herbs and garlic. Let cool slightly then cut into slices. Put into an ovenproof dish, toss with the ricotta and top with the breadcrumbs and butter. Place under the grill to melt the cheese. Serve immediately.
Serves 4.

Kitchen Pointer: Make sure not to overcook the courgettes or the whole dish will become soggy.

PER SERVING	
Kcals	89
g fat	5
g protein	5
g carbohydrate	6

Roasted New Potatoes with Herbs

In this side dish, new potatoes are perfectly offset by a delicate combination of garlic, rosemary and thyme. Serve with roast chicken, turkey or pork.

1.5 kg	new potatoes, quartered	3 lb
6 tbsp	olive oil	6 tbsp
3	cloves garlic, grated	3
1 tbsp	each dried rosemary and thyme	1 tbsp
1 tsp	dried oregano	1 tsp
	salt and pepper	

Pre-heat the oven to 230°C/450°F/Gas Mark 8.

Mix the potatoes, oil and garlic together in a bowl, and toss to coat. Add the herbs and toss again. Season with salt and pepper to taste. Divide the potatoes between two large heavy baking sheets. Bake for about 20-30 minutes or until brown and crisp, stirring occasionally.

Serves 8.

This recipe is FREE of the following triggers (marked ✔)

Caffeine ✔
Chocolate ✔
Citrus fruits ✔
Red wine ✔
Aged cheese ✔
MSG & Nitrates ✔
Aspartame ✔
Nuts ✔
Onions & Garlic
Yeast ✔

PER SERVING	
Kcals	248
g fat	12
g protein	4
g carbohydrate	31

Mushrooms and Rice

The earthy texture of rice is a perfect match with fresh mushrooms. Serve this quick-cooking side dish with your favourite grilled meats.

	basmati rice (enough for six servings)	
50 g	butter	2 oz
1	onion, finely chopped	1
2	celery stalks, finely chopped	2
350 g	mushrooms, sliced	12 oz
½ tsp	dried thyme and sage	½ tsp
	fresh parsley, chopped	
	salt and pepper	

Cook the rice in a large pan of boiling salted water. Drain and set aside to keep warm.

Melt the butter in a large frying pan over moderate heat. Add the onion and celery and fry until soft. Add the mushrooms, thyme and sage. Cook, stirring for 3-4 minutes. Add the mixture to the cooked rice, then stir in the parsley, salt and pepper to taste.

Serves 6.

PER SERVING	
Kcals	171
g fat	7
g protein	3
g carbohydrate	24

Steamed Basmati Rice with Crisp Potatoes, Sumac and Cumin

Fragrant basmati tops a layer of crisp sweet potatoes in this Middle Eastern-inspired side dish.

450 g	basmati rice	1 lb
6 tbsp	olive oil	6 tbsp
3	sweet potatoes, peeled and sliced 5 mm/¼ inch thick	3
1	lemon, pared zest only, cut in julienne strips	1
1 tbsp	each ground cumin and sumac	1 tbsp
	salt and pepper	

Cook the rice in boiling salted water for about 10 minutes or until half-cooked. Strain off the water and set aside.

Pour 2 tablespoons of the olive oil in a deep pan with a lid. Arrange the sweet potato slices side by side to cover the base of the pan. Pile the rice into the centre of the pan, making a dome shape. Push the handle of a wooden spoon into the rice several times to make air holes. Lightly drizzle rice with the remaining olive oil and season with lemon zest, cumin, sumac and salt and pepper to taste.

Cover the pan with a damp teatowel, put on the lid, then fold the edges of the teatowel over lid. Cook over moderately high heat for about 7 minutes or until the sweet potatoes are crispy.

Serve immediately.

Serves 6-8.

This recipe is FREE of the following triggers (marked ✓)
Caffeine ✓
Chocolate ✓
Citrus fruits
Red wine ✓
Aged cheese ✓
MSG & Nitrates ✓
Aspartame ✓
Nuts ✓
Onions & Garlic ✓
Yeast ✓

PER SERVING (WHEN RECIPE SERVES 8)	
Kcals	341
g fat	9
g protein	5
g carbohydrate	60

Herb and Cherry Tabbouleh

The nuttiness of bulgur is perfectly offset by the sweetness of cherries in this dish. Serve with your favourite grilled meats or as a main course salad with some bread. This salad makes an excellent addition to any picnic basket because it should be served at room temperature.

225 g	bulgur	8 oz
500 ml	boiling water or chicken stock (see p. 122)	18 fl oz
350 g	fresh cherries, stoned and halved	12 oz
2 tbsp	each chopped fresh mint and parsley	2 tbsp
	salt and pepper	
	olive oil, as needed	

Put the bulgur into a bowl, then gradually add the boiling water or chicken stock until the bulgur has swollen up and is tender, but not soggy.

Add the cherries, mint, parsley and salt and pepper to taste and mix thoroughly. Leave to stand for about 30 minutes in a cool place.

Taste and adjust the seasoning, and add more water or stock and sunflower oil, if necessary.

Serves 4-6.

Kitchen Pointer: Cherry stoners make removing the stones easier than having to cut the cherries in half and then prying the stones out.

Make Ahead: The tabbouleh can be prepared earlier in the day or a day in advance. Store in the fridge and bring to room temperature before serving.

This recipe is FREE of the following triggers (marked ✔)

Caffeine ✔
Chocolate ✔
Citrus fruits ✔
Red wine ✔
Aged cheese ✔
MSG & Nitrates ✔
Aspartame ✔
Nuts ✔
Onions & Garlic ✔
Yeast ✔

PER SERVING (WHEN RECIPE SERVES 6)	
Kcals	109
g fat	1
g protein	3
g carbohydrate	22

Bulgur and Green Bean Salad with Herbed Vinaigrette

Bulgur is parboiled cracked wheat that is easy to prepare and has a nutty flavour and pleasant chewy texture.

200 g	bulgur	7 oz
500 ml	boiling water	18 fl oz
350 g	green beans	12 oz
5 tbsp	balsamic vinegar (or cider vinegar and 1 tsp brown sugar)	5 tbsp
3	cloves garlic, crushed	3
1 tsp	each chopped fresh thyme, oregano and rosemary	1 tsp
250 ml	olive oil	9 fl oz
	salt and pepper	
3	medium tomatoes, chopped	3
100 g	chopped, stoned kalamata olives	4 oz
1	large bag mixed salad greens	1
225 g	soft mild goats' cheese, crumbled	8 oz

Combine the bulgur and water in a large bowl. Set aside.

Cook the green beans in boiling salted water in a saucepan, for about 4 minutes or until tender but crisp. Drain well and pat dry. Add to the bulgur.

Combine the vinegar, garlic and herbs then gradually whisk in the oil. Season to taste with salt and pepper.

Add the tomatoes and olives to the bulgur. Mix in enough dressing to coat completely. Season with salt and pepper to taste.

Pile the salad leaves onto a large serving platter. Top with the bulgur, then add the crumbled goats' cheese as a garnish.

Serves 6-8.

Kitchen Pointer: Chicken can be added to this dish to make a complete meal.

This recipe is FREE of the following triggers (marked ✔)

Caffeine ✔
Chocolate ✔
Citrus fruits ✔
Red wine ✔
Aged cheese ✔
MSG & Nitrates ✔
Aspartame ✔
Nuts ✔
Onions & Garlic
Yeast ✔

PER SERVING
(WHEN RECIPE SERVES 8)

Kcals	336
g fat	16
g protein	12
g carbohydrate	36

Grilled Polenta with Tomato Sauce

In this recipe, the polenta is allowed to harden and then it's sliced, grilled and served with tomato sauce to make a zesty side dish.

2	shallots, diced	2
2 tbsp	vegetable oil or butter	2 tbsp
100 g	fresh sweetcorn kernels	4 oz
1	red pepper, seeded and diced	1
1 tsp	finely chopped garlic	1 tsp
1 litre	milk	1¾ pints
1 litre	chicken stock (see p. 122)	1¾ pints
350 g	polenta	12 oz
1 tbsp	each chopped fresh mixed herbs (rosemary, thyme, etc.)	1 tbsp
½	lemon, juice from	½
	salt and pepper	
175 ml	homemade tomato sauce (or passata)	6 fl oz

Heat the oil in a large saucepan and fry the shallots until tender. Add the sweetcorn, red pepper and garlic and cook until tender.

Add the milk and chicken stock and bring to the boil over moderate heat. Slowly whisk in the polenta. Add the herbs, lemon juice and salt and pepper to taste. Cook for an additional 5-10 minutes or until creamy and thick.

Pour the polenta into a 23 cm/9 inch square cake tin, lined with clingfilm. Gently tap the tin to make sure the polenta gets into all corners. Allow to cool. Cover and chill for 2 hours (or overnight).

To serve, unmould the polenta and remove clingfilm. Cut into slices then cut on the diagonal to make triangles. Preheat the grill to high, then grill the polenta until heated through, turning once.

Heat tomato sauce until hot, then divide between individual plates. Arrange two triangles of polenta on top, per person. Garnish with sprig of fresh rosemary or thyme, if liked.

PER SERVING (WHEN RECIPE SERVES 6)	
Kcals	353
g fat	9
g protein	12
g carbohydrate	56

Serves 4-6.

Kitchen Pointer: If fresh sweetcorn is unavailable, frozen or canned can be used instead.

Make Ahead: Prepare polenta and chill up to a day in advance before grilling.

Quick Breads, Desserts and Baked Goods

Never-Fail Scones
Healthy Scones
Irish Scones
Buttermilk Scones
Corn Bread
Courgette Bread
Pancakes
Apple Pancakes
Apple Cobbler
Roasted Pears with Minted Custard
Poached Fruit in Light Syrup with Vanilla Ice Cream and Roasted Almonds
Allspice Roasted Bananas
Blueberry Maple Pie with Warmed Maple Syrup
Peach Sponge
Old-Fashioned Butterscotch Pie
Ginger Pound Cake
Maple Syrup Cake
Cranberry Carrot Cake with Cream Cheese Frosting
Crème Brûlée with Rosemary
Moltoff with Fresh Berry Compote
Lemon Curd with Shortbread and Raspberry Coulis
Mocha Mousse with Cinnamon Whipped Cream
Wholewheat Doughnuts
Carob Chip Cookies
No-Bake Carob-Oatmeal Macaroons
Almond Crescents
Ginger Snaps

Never-Fail Scones

As well as being delicious served with cream and jam, these fluffy white scones are an excellent accompaniment to stews and casseroles if you omit the sugar.

225 g	plain flour	8 oz
4 tsp	baking powder	4 tsp
1 tsp	sugar	1 tsp
½ tsp	salt	½ tsp
100 g	butter, diced	4 oz
4 tbsp	milk	4 tbsp
1	egg	1

Preheat the oven to 230°C/450°F/Gas Mark 8.

Sift the flour and baking powder together in a large bowl. Stir in the sugar and salt. Rub in the butter with your fingers. Add the milk and egg and mix to a dough. Put the dough on lightly floured surface and roll or pat out to 2 cm/¾ inch thick. Cut into rounds with a 5 cm/2 inch floured round pastry cutter.

Tranfer rounds to lightly greased baking sheet. Bake for 10-12 minutes or until lightly browned.

Makes about 8-10.

This recipe is FREE of the following triggers (marked ✔)

Caffeine ✓
Chocolate ✓
Citrus fruits ✓
Red wine ✓
Aged cheese ✓
MSG & Nitrates ✓
Aspartame ✓
Nuts ✓
Onions & Garlic ✓
Yeast ✓

PER SCONE	
Kcals	131
g fat	7
g protein	3
g carbohydrate	14

Healthy Scones

Spelt is a type of wheat. The combination of spelt and oat flour produces a surprisingly light scone with a rich, nutty flavour. This recipe can be doubled with good results.

150 g	spelt flour	5 oz
150 g	oat flour	5 oz
2 tsp	baking powder	2 tsp
1/4 tsp	bicarbonate of soda	1/4 tsp
1/4 tsp	sea salt	1/4 tsp
100 g	butter, diced	4 oz
175 ml	buttermilk	6 fl oz

Preheat the oven to 190°C/375°F/Gas Mark 5.

Combine the flours, baking powder, bicarbonate of soda and salt in a large bowl. Rub in the butter until the mixture resembles breadcrumbs. Stir in the buttermilk to form soft dough.

Turn out onto lightly floured surface and knead dough gently. Roll out to about 2 cm/3/4 inch thick and cut into rounds with a 5 cm/2 inch pastry cutter. Transfer to a lightly greased baking sheet and bake for about 10 minutes or until just golden on top.

Makes about 12.

Variations: Add chopped fresh herbs to the mix, or for sweet scones, 1 tsp sugar and 50 g/2 oz raisins or chopped candied ginger.

This recipe is FREE of the following triggers (marked ✔)

Caffeine ✔
Chocolate ✔
Citrus fruits ✔
Red wine ✔
Aged cheese ✔
MSG & Nitrates ✔
Aspartame ✔
Nuts ✔
Onions & Garlic ✔
Yeast ✔

PER SCONE	
Kcals	181
g fat	9
g protein	4
g carbohydrate	21

Irish Scones

Made with rolled oats and raisins, these scones are a nutritious and tasty alternative to ordinary scones.

275 g	plain flour	10 oz
4 tbsp	rolled oats	4 tbsp
2 tbsp	sugar	2 tbsp
2 tsp	baking powder	2 tsp
2 tsp	bicarbonate of soda	2 tsp
½ tsp	salt	½ tsp
75 g	butter	3 oz
300 ml	milk	½ pint
75 g	raisins	3 oz

Preheat the oven to 200°C/400°F/Gas Mark 6.

Mix together the flour, oats, sugar, baking powder, bicarbonate of soda and salt. With pastry blender or two knives, cut in the butter. Add the milk and stir in the raisins.

Turn the dough out onto a lightly floured surface. Pat or roll out to 2 cm/¾ inch thick. Cut into rounds using a 5 cm/2 inch pastry cutter. Bake for 10-15 minutes or until golden brown.

Makes about 12.

Kitchen Pointer: The secret to light and fluffy scones is to work the dough as little as possible. The dough toughens the more you work it because the gluten in the flour is activated.

PER SCONE	
Kcals	194
g fat	6
g protein	4
g carbohydrate	31

Buttermilk Scones

A healthy alternative to sweet scones, these can also be served as a savoury appetiser with your favourite cheese.

350 g	plain flour	12 oz
1 tbsp	baking powder	1 tbsp
1½ tsp	salt	1½ tsp
250 ml	buttermilk plus extra if needed	9 fl oz

Preheat the oven to 180°C/350°F/Gas Mark 4.

Sift the flour, baking powder and salt together in a large bowl. Gradually add enough buttermilk to make stiff dough.

Turn out onto lightly floured board and roll out to about 2 cm/¾ inch thick. Cut out rounds with a 5 cm/2 inch pastry cutter. Put on a greased baking sheet and bake for about 25 minutes or until golden brown.

Makes about 12.

This recipe is FREE of the following triggers (marked ✔)

Caffeine ✓
Chocolate ✓
Citrus fruits ✓
Red wine ✓
Aged cheese ✓
MSG & Nitrates ✓
Aspartame ✓
Nuts ✓
Onions & Garlic ✓
Yeast ✓

PER SCONE	
Kcals	129
g fat	1
g protein	4
g carbohydrate	26

Corn Bread

This corn bread is wonderful served with a large bowl of steaming beef chilli con carne.

225 g	self-raising flour	8 oz
150 g	cornmeal	5 oz
175 g	granulated sugar	6 oz
½ tsp	baking powder	½ tsp
½ tsp	salt	½ tsp
300 ml	single cream	½ pint
225 g	butter	8 oz
2	eggs, lightly beaten	2

Tip the scone mix into a large bowl and stir in the cornmeal, sugar, bicarbonate of soda and salt. Heat the cream with the butter in a saucepan then add to the dry ingredients. Mix in the eggs.

Pour the batter into a greased and floured 33 x 23 cm/ 13 x 9 inch baking dish, spreading it out evenly. Bake at 180°C/350°F/Gas Mark 4 for 30 minutes or until lightly browned and firm to the touch. Leave to stand for several minutes before cutting.
Serves 12-16.

PER SERVING	
Kcals	260
g fat	16
g protein	3
g carbohydrate	26

Courgette Bread

Rich, moist, fragrant and delicious, courgette bread is more of a treat than a bread. It's perfect for breakfast, as a snack, or for dessert.

3	eggs	3
250 g	courgettes, grated	9 oz
225 g	butter, melted	8 oz
225 g	sugar	8 oz
350 g	plain flour	12 oz
2 tsp	ground nutmeg	2 tsp
1 tsp	cinnamon	1 tsp
1 tsp	salt	1 tsp
1½ tsp	baking powder	1½ tsp

Beat the eggs together in a large bowl. Blend in the courgettes, butter and sugar.

In a separate bowl, sift the flour, nutmeg, cinnamon, salt and baking powder. Stir into the courgette mixture.

Pour the batter into two greased loaf tins (11 x 20 cm/ 4 x 8 inch). Bake at 160°C/325°F/Gas Mark 3 for 1 hour or until a skewer inserted into the centre comes out clean. Leave the loaves to cool in the tins for 10 minutes, then turn out on to rack to cool completely.

Makes 2.

Variation: Stir 100 g/4 oz raisins into the batter before pouring into loaf tins.

PER SERVING (1 SLICE)	
Kcals	135
g fat	7
g protein	2
g carbohydrate	16

Pancakes

Kids love these served with sweetened strawberries or with butter and maple syrup.

2	eggs, separated	2
175 ml	milk plus extra if necessary	6 fl oz
1 tbsp	oil	1 tbsp
100 g	plain flour	4 oz

Beat the egg whites in a large bowl until stiff. Whisk the egg yolks in another bowl until pale. Whisk in the milk then the oil to the egg yolks. Finally stir in the flour. Fold this mixture into the beaten egg whites.

Heat a large non-stick frying pan over moderate heat. Using about 4 tablespoons batter for each pancake, pour into the hot pan. When the underside is brown and bubbles break on top, turn over and fry the other side for 30 seconds or so.

Makes about 12.

PER SERVING	
Kcals	66
g fat	2
g protein	3
g carbohydrate	9

Apple Pancakes

These tasty pancakes are ideal for a special breakfast for two or three people.

170 g	plain flour	6 oz
1 tbsp	sugar	1 tbsp
1 tbsp	baking powder	1 tbsp
½ tsp	salt	½ tsp
1	egg, beaten	1
375 ml	milk	13 fl oz
2	small apples, finely chopped	2
1 tsp	cinnamon	1 tsp

Mix the flour, sugar, baking powder and salt together in a large bowl.

In a separate bowl, mix the egg and milk together then add to the dry ingredients. Stir in the apples and cinnamon.

Heat a large non-stick frying pan over moderate heat. Using about 4 tablespoons batter for each pancake, pour into the hot pan. When the underside is brown and bubbles break on top, turn over and fry the other side for 30 seconds or so. Serve with Apple Syrup (recipe below).

Makes about 12.

Apple Syrup

350 g	apples, peeled and chopped	12 oz
175 ml plus 2 tsp	apple juice	6 fl oz plus 2 tsp
100 ml	maple syrup	4 fl oz
2 tsp	cornflour	2 tsp

Combine the apples, 175 ml/6 fl oz apple juice and the maple syrup in a saucepan. Bring to the boil over moderate heat, stirring. Reduce the heat, cover and simmer for 10 minutes or until the apples are tender.

In small bowl, combine cornflour and the rest of the apple juice. Add to hot mixture and cook stirring until slightly thickened. Serve warm over apple pancakes.

This recipe is FREE of the following triggers (marked ✔)

Caffeine ✔
Chocolate ✔
Citrus fruits ✔
Red wine ✔
Aged cheese ✔
MSG & Nitrates ✔
Aspartame ✔
Nuts ✔
Onions & Garlic ✔
Yeast ✔

PER SERVING	
Kcals	97
g fat	1
g protein	3
g carbohydrate	19

Apple Cobbler

This delectable cobbler is made with rolled oats and is quick and easy to prepare. Serve it plain or with whipped cream or vanilla ice cream.

3	dessert apples, peeled and cored	3
100 ml	apple juice	4 fl oz
50 g	granulated sugar	2 oz
1 tbsp	cinnamon	1 tbsp
1 tsp	nutmeg	1 tsp
75 g	uncooked rolled oats	3 oz
225 g	brown sugar	8 oz
50 g	plain flour	2 oz
100 g	unsalted butter	4 oz

Cut the apples into 5 mm/¼ inch slices.

Put into a small saucepan with the apple juice, granulated sugar, cinnamon and nutmeg.

Cook over moderate heat for about 10 minutes, stirring occasionally, or until the mixture becomes syrupy.

Mix the rolled oats, brown sugar and flour. Rub in the butter until the mixture looks like coarse breadcrumbs.

Pour the apple mixture into a 10 cm/4 inch deep baking dish and top evenly with the oat mixture. Bake at 200°C/400°F/Gas Mark 6 for about 4-5 minutes or until the topping is browned and the fruit is bubbling.

Serves 2-4.

Make Ahead: The cobbler can be prepared several hours ahead and kept at room temperature before baking.

This recipe is FREE of the following triggers (marked ✔)

Caffeine ✔
Chocolate ✔
Citrus fruits ✔
Red wine ✔
Aged cheese ✔
MSG & Nitrates ✔
Aspartame ✔
Nuts ✔
Onions & Garlic ✔
Yeast ✔

PER SERVING
(WHEN RECIPE SERVES 4)

Kcals	706
g fat	26
g protein	6
g carbohydrate	112

Roasted Pears with Minted Custard

Serve this elegant dessert decorated with fresh mint or with a scoop of your favourite ice cream.

225 g	granulated sugar	8 oz
250 ml	water	9 fl oz
4	pears, firm but ripe	4
Sauce		
8	egg yolks	8
225 g	caster sugar	8 oz
2 tsp	cornflour (optional)	2 tsp
1 litre	skimmed milk	1¾ pints
1	bunch fresh mint, chopped	1
	extra mint to decorate	

Combine the sugar and water in a heavy-based saucepan. Bring to the boil then boil for several minutes only. Remove from heat and allow to cool. This makes a simple syrup.

Peel and core pears. Wrap the stems in foil (to stop them burning). Cut the pears into slices, keeping them joined at the stem end (so the pears will fan out on plate). Dip the pears into the syrup. Arrange the pears on a greased baking sheet and cook at 200°C/400°F/Gas Mark 6 for about 30 minutes or until browned.

Sauce
Whisk the egg yolks and sugar together in a bowl and beat in the cornflour, if using. Set aside.

Heat the milk and mint together in a saucepan over moderate heat, stirring occasionally. Bring the milk up to boiling point, stirring often, but do not boil. Strain the milk into a jug. Gradually add to the egg yolk mixture, in a thin stream, whisking all the time.

Pour the sauce into the top of a double boiler or into a bowl, set over a saucepan of simmering water. Cook the sauce, stirring constantly, until it coats the back of the spoon. Remove from heat and leave to cool. To serve, spoon some custard onto dessert plates. Fan out a warm caramelized pear on each plate. Decorate with fresh mint.
Serves 4.

Make Ahead: The custard may be made up to two days in advance and stored in the fridge.

This recipe is FREE of the following triggers (marked ✔)

Caffeine ✔
Chocolate ✔
Citrus fruits ✔
Red wine ✔
Aged cheese ✔
MSG & Nitrates ✔
Aspartame ✔
Nuts ✔
Onions & Garlic ✔
Yeast ✔

PER SERVING (1 PEAR WITH 50 ML/2 FL OZ SAUCE)

Kcals	225
g fat	5
g protein	4
g carbohydrate	41

Poached Fruit in Light Syrup with Vanilla Ice Cream and Roasted Almonds

Vary the fruit in this recipe to suit the season. This elegant and tasty dessert is sure to impress your guests.

450 g	granulated sugar	1 lb
1 litre	water	1³/₄ pints
1	pear, cut into wedges	1
1	peach, cut into wedges	1
170 g	fresh strawberries, hulled	6 oz
8	scoops good quality vanilla ice cream	8
50 g	slivered toasted almonds	2 oz

Combine the sugar and water in heavy-based pan. Bring to the boil and boil gently, stirring occasionally, for 5 minutes.

Add the pear wedges to the syrup and cook for 1 minute. Remove pear wedges. Add the peach wedges to syrup and cook for 10 seconds, then remove these. Add the strawberries to the syrup for 10 seconds and remove from the syrup.

Continue to boil the syrup until it thickens.

Meanwhile, alternate layers of fruit and ice cream in four champagne flutes. Top with slivered toasted almonds. Using a tablespoon, drizzle some of syrup over the almonds. Serve immediately.

Serves 4.

PER SERVING	
Kcals	380
g fat	16
g protein	4
g carbohydrate	55

Allspice Roasted Bananas

A simple but tasty dessert, perfect with vanilla ice cream.

8	bananas, small to medium	8
100 g	brown sugar	4 oz
100 g	unsalted butter, melted	4 oz
5	whole allspice	5

Peel the bananas and arrange in a baking dish. Sprinkle with brown sugar then drizzle with melted butter. Scatter allspice over the top.

Bake at 220°C/425°F/Gas Mark 7 for about 10 minutes or until the sugar melts, bubbles and caramelises. Serve with vanilla ice cream or yogurt.

Serves 6-8.

Kitchen Pointer: Watch carefully as the sugar may burn if left too long.

This recipe is FREE of the following triggers (marked ✔)

Caffeine ✓
Chocolate ✓
Citrus fruits ✓
Red wine ✓
Aged cheese ✓
MSG & Nitrates ✓
Aspartame ✓
Nuts ✓
Onions & Garlic ✓
Yeast ✓

PER SERVING
(WHEN RECIPE SERVES 8)

Kcals	352
g fat	10
g protein	0.4
g carbohydrate	19

Blueberry Maple Pie with Warmed Maple Syrup

Maple syrup adds a delectable touch to this blueberry pie that's perfect with vanilla ice cream.

Pastry		
125 ml	cold water	4 fl oz
pinch	salt	pinch
1 tbsp	maple syrup	1 tbsp
175 g	cold vegetable fat	6 oz
350 g	plain flour	12 oz
1	egg, beaten	1
Filling		
675 g	fresh or frozen blueberries	1 1/4 lb
100 g	granulated sugar	4 oz
4 tbsp	maple syrup	4 tbsp
2 tbsp	cornflour	2 tbsp
1/4 tsp	cinnamon	1/4 tsp

This recipe is FREE of the following triggers (marked ✔)

Caffeine ✔
Chocolate ✔
Citrus fruits ✔
Red wine ✔
Aged cheese ✔
MSG & Nitrates ✔
Aspartame ✔
Nuts ✔
Onions & Garlic ✔
Yeast ✔

Pastry

Pour the water into a bowl, and stir in the salt and maple syrup. In a large mixing bowl or food processor, rub the vegetable fat into the flour until mixture resembles coarse breadcrumb. Make a well in the centre and gradually add enough of the water mixture, to make a dough. Knead dough very lightly and form into ball. Wrap in clingfilm and chill for at least 30 minutes or overnight.

Filling

Cut the dough into two pieces, one slightly larger than the other. On a lightly floured surface, roll out the larger piece of dough to fit a 23 cm/9 inch pie tin with a slight overhang. Roll out the second piece of dough for the lid.

Line the bottom of pie tin with dough and gently press into place. Combine the blueberries, sugar, maple syrup, cornflour and cinnamon and spoon into pastry-lined tin.

Cover with the pastry lid. Press the edges together then trim off excess pastry. Brush with beaten egg.

Make several slits in dough to allow steam to escape. Bake at 190°C/375°F/Gas Mark 5 for 30-35 minutes until the pastry is golden.

PER SERVING	
Kcals	480
g fat	28
g protein	4
g carbohydrate	53

Serve warm or at room temperature with vanilla ice cream topped with warmed maple syrup.

Serves 8.

Make Ahead: Prepare the pastry a day in advance. The pie can be baked earlier in the day and then warmed just before serving.

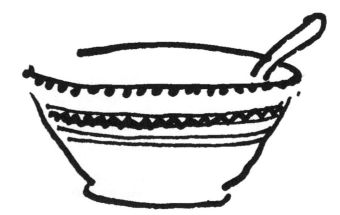

Peach Sponge

Peaches, artfully arranged on top of a sponge cake and baked in the oven, make an impressive dessert for entertaining. Try serving this with a dollop of whipped cream.

100 g	butter	4 oz
100 g	caster sugar plus 4 tbsp	4 oz
100 g	self-raising flour	4 oz
1 tsp	baking powder	1 tsp
pinch	salt	pinch
2	eggs	2
4	peaches, sliced	4
3 tbsp	lemon juice	3 tbsp
pinch	each cinnamon and nutmeg	pinch

Cream the butter and sugar together in a large bowl. Add the flour, baking powder and salt. Add the eggs and beat well.

Scrape the batter into a greased and lined 20 cm/8 inch cake tin. Arrange the peaches, skin side up, in a pattern on the top.

Sprinkle with the rest of the sugar and the lemon juice, cinnamon, and nutmeg.

Bake in 180°C/350°F/Gas Mark 4 for 1 hour or until the peaches are tender and the cake is risen and golden.

Serves 8-10.

PER SERVING (WHEN RECIPE SERVES 10)	
Kcals	243
g fat	11
g protein	3
g carbohydrate	33

Old-Fashioned Butterscotch Pie

No one can resist the rich buttery goodness of this wonderful dessert.

1	baked 23 cm/9 inch pastry case (see pastry recipe page 94, use half quantity)	1
175 g	brown sugar	6 oz
2 tbsp	plain flour	2 tbsp
425 ml	milk (half evaporated)	¾ pint
15 g	butter	½ oz
2	egg yolks, well beaten	2
1 tsp	vanilla extract	1 tsp

Mix the sugar and flour together in a saucepan, then stir in the milk.

Cook the mixture over moderate heat until thickened.

Remove from the heat, then add the butter and egg yolks. Return to the heat and cook for 2 minutes longer. Remove from the heat.

Stir in the vanilla then pour the mixture into pastry case. Top with meringue (recipe follows).

Meringue for Butterscotch Pie

2	egg whites	2
100 g	caster sugar	4 oz

Beat the egg whites in a bowl until soft peaks form. Very gradually beat in the sugar until mixture is stiff and glossy. Spread evenly over the filling. Bake at 220°C/425°F/Gas Mark 7 for 4-5 minutes or until the tips of the meringue are golden. Leave to cool, then chill before serving.
Serves 8.

PER SERVING	
Kcals	288
g fat	12
g protein	6
g carbohydrate	39

Ginger Pound Cake

Ginger adds a unique taste to this simple and delicious cake.

225 g	butter	8 oz
225 g	caster sugar	8 oz
4	eggs	4
1 tsp	vanilla extract	1 tsp
225 g	self-raising flour	8 oz
½ tsp	baking powder	½ tsp
¼ tsp	salt	¼ tsp
350 g	ginger marmalade	12 oz

Cream the butter with the sugar in a mixing bowl until light and fluffy. Add the eggs one at a time, beating well after each. Beat in the vanilla.

In a separate bowl, combine the flour, baking powder and salt. Fold the flour mixture into butter mixture, then stir in the marmalade.

Turn the batter into a greased and floured 23 x 12.5 cm/ 9 x 5 inch loaf tin. Bake at 160°C/325°F/Gas Mark 3 for about 1¼-1½ hours or until a skewer comes out clean. Leave to cool in the tin, then turn out onto a rack to cool completely.

Serves 8-12.

PER SERVING (WHEN RECIPE SERVES 12)	
Kcals	426
g fat	18
g protein	5
g carbohydrate	61

Maple Syrup Cake

Toasted coconut adds a delightful crunchiness to this moist maple cake.

Sauce

250 ml	maple syrup	9 fl oz
175 ml	water	6 fl oz
2 tsp	butter	2 tsp

Cake

100 g	self-raising flour	4 oz
100 g	caster sugar	4 oz
1½ tsp	baking powder	1½ tsp
½ tsp	salt	½ tsp
1	egg, well beaten	1
75 ml	milk	3 fl oz
15 g	vegetable fat	½ oz
50 g	shredded coconut	2 oz
	whipped cream	

Bring the syrup and water to boil in a saucepan. Remove from the heat and stir in the butter. Set aside.

Mix the flour, sugar, baking powder and salt together in a large bowl. Beat in the egg, milk and vegetable fat to make a batter. Pour into a greased 20 cm/8 inch square cake tin.

Pour the maple syrup sauce slowly over the batter. Sprinkle the coconut on top. Bake at 180°C/350°F/Gas Mark 4 for 35 minutes or until a skewer inserted in the centre comes out clean. Cool on a wire rack. Serve with whipped cream.

Serves 8-12.

PER SERVING (WHEN RECIPE SERVES 12)	
Kcals	220
g fat	4
g protein	3
g carbohydrate	43

Cranberry Carrot Cake with Cream Cheese Frosting

The cranberries in this recipe add a subtle tartness to this perennial favourite.

350 g	granulated sugar	12 oz
250 ml	vegetable oil	9 fl oz
5	eggs, at room temperature	5
275 g	plain flour	10 oz
2¼ tsp	baking powder	2¼ tsp
2¼ tsp	cinnamon	2¼ tsp
2 tsp	bicarbonate of soda	2 tsp
1 tsp	salt	1 tsp
350 g	carrots, peeled and grated	12 oz
175 g	fresh cranberries	6 oz

Combine the sugar, oil and eggs in a large mixing bowl.
Add the flour, baking powder, cinnamon, bicarbonate of soda and salt and mix together. Fold in the carrots and cranberries. Divide evenly between two 23 cm/9 inch round greased and floured cake tins.
Bake at 150°C/300°F/Gas Mark 2 for about 45 minutes or until a skewer inserted in the centre comes out clean.
Cool for 10 minutes in the tins before turning out onto racks to cool completely. When cold, cover with Cream Cheese Frosting (recipe follows).

Cream Cheese Frosting

100 g	unsalted butter, at room temperature	4 oz
225 g	cream cheese	8 oz
1 tsp	vanilla extract	1 tsp
600 g	icing sugar	1 lb 5 oz
¼ tsp	grated lemon zest	¼ tsp

This recipe is FREE of the following triggers (marked ✔)

Caffeine ✔
Chocolate ✔
Citrus fruits
Red wine ✔
Aged cheese ✔
MSG & Nitrates ✔
Aspartame ✔
Nuts ✔
Onions & Garlic ✔
Yeast ✔

PER SERVING
(WHEN RECIPE SERVES 16)

Kcals	551
g fat	27
g protein	6
g carbohydrate	71

Cream the butter, cream cheese and vanilla extract until fluffy. Beat in icing sugar until the frosting is smooth and spreadable. Stir in the lemon zest. Spread over the cake.

Serves 12-16.

Make Ahead: The Cranberry Carrot Cake can be baked a day in advance, wrapped in clingfilm or foil, and stored at room temperature until ready to be covered with frosting.

Crème Brûlée with Rosemary

This traditional French recipe is brought up to date with the addition of fragrant rosemary.

6	egg yolks, at room temperature	6
75 g	caster sugar	3 oz
500 ml	whipping cream	18 fl oz
100 ml	milk	4 fl oz
1 tbsp	chopped fresh rosemary	1 tbsp
	granulated sugar for caramelising	

Whisk the egg yolks and sugar together in a bowl until well blended.

Bring the cream, milk and rosemary to gentle boil in a heavy-based saucepan, stirring occasionally. Remove from the heat.

Gradually pour the heated cream mixture onto the egg yolks and sugar, constantly beating with whisk. Leave the mixture to sit for 30 minutes at room temperature.

Strain the mixture through a sieve into ramekins. Place ramekins in a roasting pan. Fill the pan with boiling water so that it comes half-way up sides of the ramekins.

Bake at 180°C/350°F/Gas Mark 4 for 30 minutes until firm. Remove the ramekins from the roasting pan and leave to cool. When cold, chill in the fridge.

Just before serving, cover the custard with a generous layer of granulated sugar. Caramelise by placing ramekins on a baking sheet and putting under a hot grill. Watch carefully and remove once the sugar has turned to a rich amber colour.

Serves 4.

This recipe is FREE of the following triggers (marked ✔)

Caffeine ✔
Chocolate ✔
Citrus fruits ✔
Red wine ✔
Aged cheese ✔
MSG & Nitrates ✔
Aspartame ✔
Nuts ✔
Onions & Garlic ✔
Yeast ✔

PER SERVING	
Kcals	580
g fat	52
g protein	8
g carbohydrate	20

Right:
Courgette Bread (page 87)

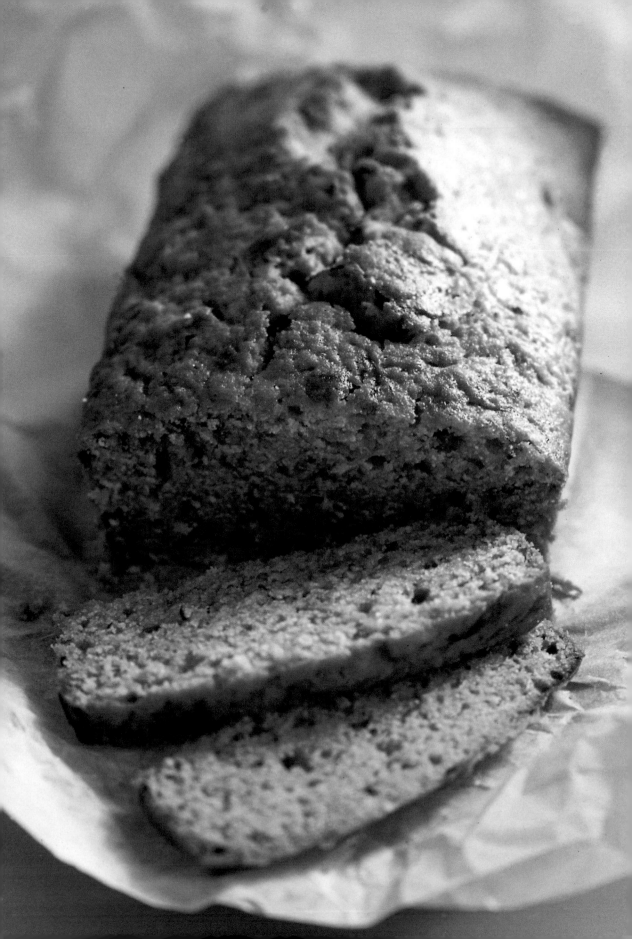

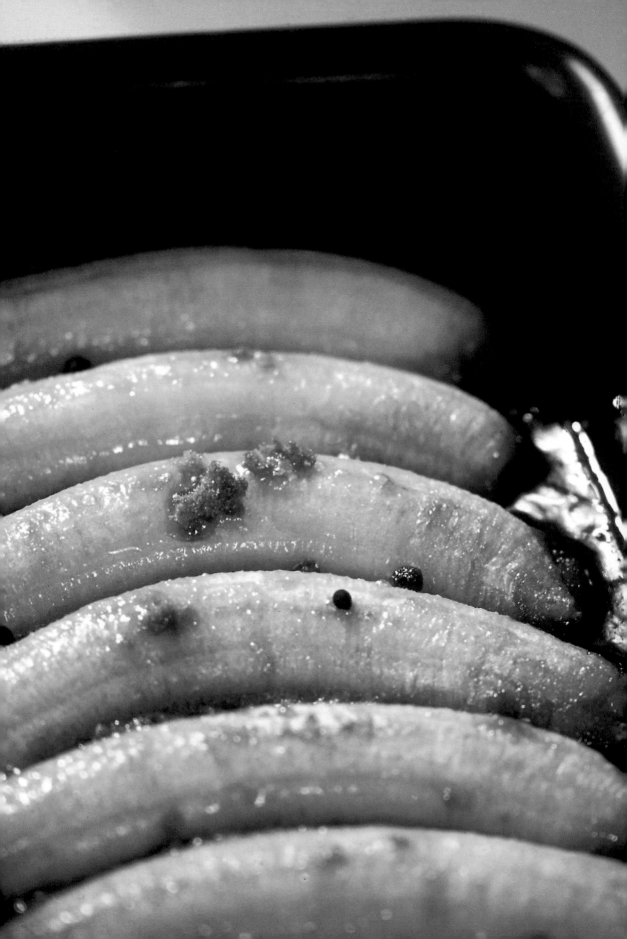

Moltoff with Fresh Berry Compote

This fantastically light and elegant dessert will leave your guests clamouring for more!

Caramel Moltoff

675 g	granulated sugar	1½ lb
250 ml	water	9 fl oz
10	egg whites	10
250 g	caster sugar	9 oz
1 tsp	baking powder	1 tsp
25 g	unsalted butter	1 oz
300 ml	vanilla custard, bought or homemade, for serving	½ pint

   Melt the granulated sugar in a small heavy-based saucepan, stirring until darkened in colour. Add the water and leave to reduce to the syrup stage. Do not allow to reduce too much as it will thicken slightly as it cools.
Beat the egg whites with the caster sugar and baking powder until soft peaks form. Beat in 1 tablespoon of caramel.
Set the remaining caramel aside for serving. Butter the inside of a chilled round angel cake tin and fill with the egg white mixture. Place the filled pan in a deep roasting pan containing enough boiling water to come halfway up sides of the cake tin.
   Bake at 190°C/375°F/Gas Mark 5 for 10-14 minutes or until golden brown. Remove from oven and water bath and leave to cool to room temperature. Invert onto rack and remove from pan.

Fresh Berry Compote

250 ml	water	9 fl oz
500 g	granulated sugar	18 oz
2 tbsp	orange liqueur (optional)	2 tbsp
225 g	each fresh blueberries, raspberries and strawberries	8 oz
	icing sugar	

PER SERVING (WHEN RECIPE SERVES 10)	
Kcals	399
g fat	3
g protein	5
g carbohydrate	88

Left:
Allspice Roasted Bananas
(page 93)

Bring the water, sugar and orange liqueur (if using) to the boil over moderately high heat in a heavy-based saucepan. Simmer until the mixture becomes syrup. Add the berries and remove from the heat. Leave to cool to room temperature.

Reheat the remaining caramel. Pour a little custard onto individual dessert plates. Slice moltoff into sections and place on top of the custard. Top with berry compote and drizzle with reheated caramel. Dust edge of each plate with some sifted icing sugar.

Serves 8-10.

Make Ahead: The moltoff, caramel and berry compote can all be made a day in advance. Chill overnight and bring to room temperature before serving.

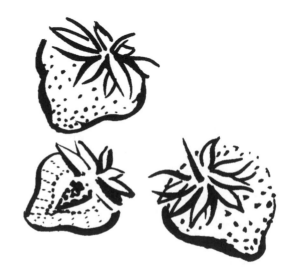

Lemon Curd with Shortbread and Raspberry Coulis

The sweetness of the shortbread and the raspberries is matched with the zesty taste of lemon in this delectable recipe.

Lemon Curd

4	egg yolks, at room temperature	4
100 g	granulated sugar	4 oz
75 ml	fresh lemon juice	3 fl oz
50 g	unsalted butter, at room temperature	2 oz
pinch	salt	pinch
2 tsp	lemon zest	2 tsp

Whisk the egg yolks and sugar together in a small heavy-based saucepan.

Add the lemon juice, butter and salt.

Cook over moderately low heat, stirring constantly until the mixture has thickened. Do not boil.

Spoon the lemon zest into a bowl, and strain the egg mixture onto it.

Leave the curd to cool then store covered in the fridge if not using straight away.

Raspberry Coulis

125 ml	water	4 fl oz
1 tbsp	cornflour	1 tbsp
1	pkt (about 425 g/15 oz) frozen raspberries	1

Mix the water and cornflour together in a bowl.

Simmer the raspberries in a saucepan over moderate heat until softened, add a little sugar to taste if desired. Quickly bring to boil, then add the cornflour and water mixture, stirring constantly.

Cook for 1 minute, stirring constantly. Don't cook too long or it will turn brown.

Remove from the heat and leave to cool.

Shortbread

350 g	unsalted butter, at room temperature	12 oz
100 g	granulated sugar	4 oz
450 g	plain flour, sifted 3 times	1 lb

Cream the butter and sugar together in a mixing bowl until very light and fluffy.

Gradually add the flour, kneading it in at the end. On a lightly floured surface, pat the dough out into a circle, then roll out to 5 mm/¼ inch thickness.

Cut into 10 cm/4 inch circles. Gather scraps, re-roll and cut into as many circles as possible.

Place the shortbread on baking sheets lined with waxed paper. Bake at 180°C/350°F/Gas Mark 4 for 10-12 minutes or until lightly golden. Transfer to a rack to cool.

Place a piece of shortbread on each plate. Top with 1 tablespoon lemon curd then some raspberry coulis. Decorate with fresh raspberries or blueberries if liked.

Serves 6-8.

Make Ahead: Lemon curd can be prepared a day in advance, raspberry coulis can be prepared several days in advance, and the shortbread a day or two in advance. Store them individually in airtight containers in the fridge.

Mocha Mousse with Cinnamon Whipped Cream

This rich dessert is quickly assembled. It contains decaffeinated espresso, but, even 'decaffeinated' coffees contain small amounts of caffeine.

5	eggs, at room temperature, separated	5
225 g	caster sugar	8 oz
100 g	unsalted butter, melted	4 oz
175 ml	decaffeinated espresso (or instant)	6 fl oz
500 ml	whipping cream	18 fl oz

Beat the egg yolks and sugar in a bowl placed over a pan of simmering water, or in the top part of a double boiler. Whisk in the butter. Cook, whisking constantly, for 6-8 minutes or until the mixture is thick, like custard. Don't overcook the eggs or allow the water to boil or the eggs will curdle.

Remove from the heat and stir in the espresso. Leave to go cold.

Beat the egg whites in a large bowl until stiff peaks form. Whip cream until stiff. Gently fold egg whites into whipped cream.

Stir about one third of the egg-cream mixture into the cold coffee mixture until thoroughly mixed, then fold in the rest. Pour into eight dessert dishes or martini glasses. Chill for several hours. Serve with Cinnamon Whipped Cream (recipe follows).

Cinnamon Whipped Cream

3 tbsp	granulated sugar	3 tbsp
1 tsp	cinnamon	1 tsp
250 ml	whipping cream	9 fl oz

Mix the sugar and cinnamon together in a small bowl. Whip the cream in a large bowl until frothy. Add the sugar mixture and whip until peaks just start to form. Serve on top of mocha mousse.

Serves 8.

Make Ahead: The Mocha Mousse can be made earlier in the day and chilled for several hours.

This recipe is FREE of the following triggers (marked ✔)

Caffeine
Chocolate ✔
Citrus fruits ✔
Red wine ✔
Aged cheese ✔
MSG & Nitrates ✔
Aspartame ✔
Nuts ✔
Onions & Garlic ✔
Yeast ✔

PER SERVING	
Kcals	420
g fat	32
g protein	5
g carbohydrate	28

Wholewheat Doughnuts

The wholewheat flour in these doughnuts adds a nice texture. They're great for dunking in coffee or tea.

275 g	plain flour	10 oz
275 g	wholewheat flour	10 oz
2 tsp	each bicarbonate of soda, baking powder and cream of tartar	2 tsp
3	eggs	3
350 g	caster sugar	12 oz
1 tsp	vanilla extract	1 tsp
1 tsp	nutmeg	1 tsp
1 tsp	salt	1 tsp
½ tsp	ground ginger	½ tsp
50 g	butter	2 oz
350 ml	milk	12 fl oz
	vegetable oil for frying	
	sugar and cinnamon for rolling (optional)	

Mix the flours, bicarbonate of soda, baking powder and cream of tartar together in a large bowl. Set aside.

In another large bowl, beat the eggs, sugar, vanilla, nutmeg, salt and ginger together until thick.

Melt the butter and add to the milk. Add milk mixture alternately with flour mixture to egg mixture, beating well after each addition. Cover dough and chill for at least 2 hours or overnight.

Tear off pieces of dough and with floured hands, roll into about 48 balls. Deep-fry at 190°C/375°F until golden brown on both sides. Drain on kitchen paper, then roll in sugar and cinnamon mixture if liked.

Makes 48.

PER DOUGHNUT	
Kcals	211
g fat	15
g protein	2
g carbohydrate	17

Carob Chip Cookies

If chocolate is a trigger, try these delectable carob chip cookies. Kids – and adults – love them.

175 g	plain flour	6 oz
2 tsp	baking powder	2 tsp
½ tsp	bicarbonate of soda	½ tsp
½ tsp	salt	½ tsp
175 g	brown sugar	6 oz
100 g	butter	4 oz
1	egg	1
75 ml	golden syrup	3 fl oz
1 tsp	vanilla extract (optional)	1 tsp
170 g	carob chips	6 oz

Sift the flour, baking powder, bicarbonate of soda and salt together in a large mixing bowl.

In another bowl, cream the sugar, butter, egg, golden syrup and vanilla together. Fold in the sifted dry ingredients then add the carob chips, mixing gently with your fingers.

Drop teaspoonfuls of the mixture well apart on to greased baking sheets. Bake at 180°C/350°F/Gas Mark 4 for 10-12 minutes or until golden brown. Cool on the baking sheet for a few minutes, then transfer to racks to cool completely.

Makes about 60.

PER COOKIE	
Kcals	63
g fat	3
g protein	1
g carbohydrate	8

No-Bake Carob-Oatmeal Macaroons

These yummy treats can be ready in less than 15 minutes.

450 g	granulated sugar	1 lb
100 g	vegetable fat	4 oz
50 g	carob powder	2 oz
125 ml	milk (or milk substitute)	4 fl oz
250 g	rolled oats	9 oz
75 g	shredded coconut or raisins	3 oz

Mix the sugar, vegetable fat, carob powder and milk together in a large saucepan. Bring the mixture to the boil. Remove from the heat and add the oats and coconut (or raisins). Mix well and drop tablespoonfuls on to baking sheets lined with with waxed paper. Leave to cool and harden.
Makes about 36.

This recipe is FREE of the following triggers (marked ✔)

Caffeine ✔
Chocolate ✔
Citrus fruits ✔
Red wine ✔
Aged cheese ✔
MSG & Nitrates ✔
Aspartame ✔
Nuts ✔
Onions & Garlic ✔
Yeast ✔

PER MACAROON	
Kcals	112
g fat	4
g protein	1
g carbohydrate	18

Almond Crescents

These crescent-shaped treats have the mellow flavour of almonds and icing sugar. They're perfect with herbal tea.

250 g	flour	9 oz
½ tsp	salt	½ tsp
275 g	softened butter	10 oz
150 g	icing sugar plus extra for dusting	5 oz
2 tsp	vanilla extract	2 tsp
100 g	ground almonds	4 oz

Mix the flour and salt together in a bowl. In a separate bowl, cream the butter with the sugar then stir in the vanilla. Gradually add the dry ingredients to the creamed mixture, then add the almonds.

Roll into 2.5 cm/1 inch balls then shape into crescents. Bake at 160°C/325°F/Gas Mark 3 on ungreased baking sheets, for 12-15 minutes or until lightly browned. Dust with icing sugar while still warm.

Makes about 72.

This recipe is FREE of the following triggers (marked ✔)

Caffeine ✔
Chocolate ✔
Citrus fruits ✔
Red wine ✔
Aged cheese ✔
MSG & Nitrates ✔
Aspartame ✔
Nuts
Onions & Garlic ✔
Yeast ✔

PER CRESCENT	
Kcals	64
g fat	4
g protein	1
g carbohydrate	6

Ginger Snaps

Memories of childhood will abound when the warm and wonderful aroma of baking ginger snaps fills your kitchen.

225 g	vegetable fat	8 oz
150 ml	molasses	5 fl oz
75 g	brown sugar	3 oz
350 g	plain flour	12 oz
2 tsp	ground ginger	2 tsp
1 tsp	cinnamon	1 tsp
½ tsp	salt	½ tsp
½ tsp	bicarbonate of soda	½ tsp
½ tsp	ground cloves	½ tsp

Cream the vegetable fat, molasses and brown sugar together in a bowl. In a separate bowl, mix the flour, ginger, cinnamon, salt, bicarbonate of soda and cloves. Add to the creamed mixture and mix to a dough. Shape the dough into a roll about 5 cm/2 inches in diameter. Wrap in waxed paper and chill for about 4 hours or until firm.

Cut the dough into 5 mm/¼ inch slices. Bake on greased baking sheets at 200°C/400°F/Gas Mark 6 for 5-7 minutes or until lightly browned. Leave to cool for a few minutes on baking sheets then transfer to racks to cool completely.

Makes about 60.

PER GINGER SNAP	
Kcals	72
g fat	4
g protein	1
g carbohydrate	8

Beverages

Mint Julep

Peppermint Cooler

Migraine Mellower

Fruit Punch

Hot Spiced Punch

Mulled Cider

Mint Julep

On a warm summer's evening, this sweet but tangy drink from America's Deep South is the perfect refresher. Substitute apple juice for the lemon juice if citrus is a trigger.

1	bunch fresh mint	1
350 g	sugar	12 oz
250 ml	lemon juice	9 fl oz
150 ml	water	¼ pint
1.7 litres	ginger ale	3 pints

Discard the stems and any bruised mint leaves. Put the good leaves into a large bowl and add the sugar, lemon juice and water. Leave to stand for 30 minutes. Fill a large jug with ice then pour over the julep. Top up with ginger ale.
Serves 10.

This recipe is FREE of the following triggers (marked ✓)

Caffeine ✓
Chocolate ✓
Citrus fruits
Red wine ✓
Aged cheese ✓
MSG & Nitrates ✓
Aspartame ✓
Nuts ✓
Onions & Garlic ✓
Yeast ✓

PER SERVING	
Kcals	176
g carbohydrate	44

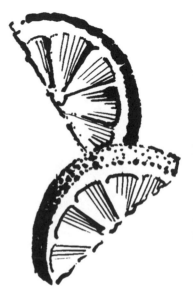

Peppermint Cooler

This frosty drink is excellent served as a dessert. It's rich in calcium, too!

2 litres	milk	3½ pints
100 g	sugar	4 oz
1 tsp	peppermint extract (or more to taste)	1 tsp
	vanilla ice cream	
	mint leaves	

Heat the milk and sugar in a large saucepan, until the sugar has dissolved. Leave to cool then chill in the fridge.

Add the peppermint extract. To serve, place a scoop of vanilla ice cream in a tall glass and pour the milk mixture over it. Decorate with mint leaves.

Serves 8.

This recipe is FREE of the following triggers (marked ✔)

Caffeine ✔
Chocolate ✔
Citrus fruits ✔
Red wine ✔
Aged cheese ✔
MSG & Nitrates ✔
Aspartame ✔
Nuts ✔
Onions & Garlic ✔
Yeast ✔

PER SERVING	
Kcals	261
g fat	9
g protein	10
g carbohydrate	35

Migraine Mellower

A soothing drink with the medicinal attributes of ginger.

75 ml	apple juice	3 fl oz
100 ml	ginger ale or ginger beer	4 fl oz

Pour the apple juice and ginger ale into a tall glass and give it a mix. Decorate with a thin slice of stem ginger, if liked.
Serves 1.

This recipe is FREE of the following triggers (marked ✔)

Caffeine ✔
Chocolate ✔
Citrus fruits ✔
Red wine ✔
Aged cheese ✔
MSG & Nitrates ✔
Aspartame ✔
Nuts ✔
Onions & Garlic ✔
Yeast ✔

PER SERVING

Kcals	80
g carbohydrate	20

Fruit Punch

Try making a frozen version of this punch. Your children will love this delicious slushy treat.

350 ml	unsweetened apple juice concentrate	12 fl oz
350 ml	unsweetened grape juice	12 fl oz
75 ml	fresh squeezed lemon juice	3 fl oz
50 ml	cranberry juice (optional)	2 fl oz
1 litre	soda water	1¾ pints

Stir the apple juice concentrate, grape juice, lemon juice and cranberry juice if using, in a large bowl. Add the soda water and stir to mix.

Kitchen Pointer: Fill a sealable plastic beaker with some of this then freeze it. Added to your child's lunch box, it'll keep everything cool until it's time to eat, and double up as a drink.

This recipe is FREE of the following triggers (marked ✔)

Caffeine ✔
Chocolate ✔
Citrus fruits
Red wine ✔
Aged cheese ✔
MSG & Nitrates ✔
Aspartame ✔
Nuts ✔
Onions & Garlic ✔
Yeast ✔

PER SERVING
(250 ML/9FL OZ)

Kcals	120
g carbohydrate	30

Hot Spiced Punch

In winter, welcome guests with this special warming drink.

500 ml	cranberry juice	18 fl oz
2 litres	apple juice	3½ pints
2	cinnamon sticks	2
6	whole cloves	6
100 g	brown sugar	4 oz

    Pour the cranberry juice, apple juice, cinnamon sticks, cloves and sugar into a large saucepan. Bring to a gentle boil, then reduce the heat and simmer for about 5 minutes. **Serves 10.**

This recipe is FREE of the following triggers (marked ✔)

Caffeine ✔
Chocolate ✔
Citrus fruits ✔
Red wine ✔
Aged cheese ✔
MSG & Nitrates ✔
Aspartame ✔
Nuts ✔
Onions & Garlic ✔
Yeast ✔

PER SERVING
(250 ML/9FL OZ)

Kcals	172
g carbohydrate	43

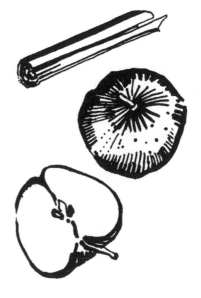

Mulled Cider

This old-fashioned favourite is perfect for a festive Christmas gathering or wintry night in with the family.

This recipe is FREE of the following triggers (marked ✔)

Caffeine ✔
Chocolate ✔
Citrus fruits ✔
Red wine ✔
Aged cheese ✔
MSG & Nitrates ✔
Aspartame ✔
Nuts ✔
Onions & Garlic ✔
Yeast ✔

1	large apple	1
20	cloves	20
1 litre	apple juice or apple cider	1¾ pints
½	whole nutmeg	½
5	short cinnamon sticks (4 for garnish)	5
1 tsp	ground ginger	1 tsp
175 g	brown sugar	6 oz

Stud the apple with the cloves. Put into a saucepan and pour in the apple juice. Add the nutmeg, one cinnamon stick and the ginger. Simmer for 30 minutes. Add the sugar, then strain into mugs. Garnish each mug with a cinnamon stick and a slice of apple.

Serves 4.

PER SERVING

Kcals	280
g carbohydrate	70

Basic Stocks and Sauces

Vegetable Stock

Chicken or Beef Stock

Fish Stock

Hollandaise Sauce

Homemade Soy Sauce

Vegetable Stock

Here's a flavourful meatless stock that will keep in the fridge for one week or can be frozen for later use.

1 tbsp	olive oil	1 tbsp
450 g	carrots, sliced	1 lb
2	large onions, sliced	2
2	leeks, sliced	2
3	celery stalks, sliced	3
100 g	parsnips, peeled, cored and sliced	4 oz
1	small bunch parsley sprigs	1
3	cloves garlic	3
2	fresh thyme sprigs	2
2 tbsp	chopped fresh basil	2 tbsp
1	bay leaf	1
1 tsp	whole black peppercorns	1 tsp
2 tsp	sea salt	2 tsp
1	medium potato, sliced	1
2	medium tomatoes, chopped	2
3 litres	water	5 pints

Heat the olive oil in a large deep saucepan over moderately high heat. Add all the ingredients except the potato, tomatoes and water. Cook, stirring occasionally, for about 6-8 minutes or until the vegetables soften.

Add the potato, tomatoes and water. Bring to the boil, reduce the heat and simmer, covered, for 40 minutes. Strain the stock over a bowl, pressing down on vegetables to extract as much stock as possible.

Leave to go cold, cover tightly with clingfilm and chill.
Makes 3 litres/5 pints.

NUTRIENTS

Contains less than 10 calories per 250 ml/9 fl oz and trace amounts of protein, fat and carbohydrates.

Chicken or Beef Stock

Canned soups and stock cubes often contain MSG or other preservatives that can be triggers. Fortunately, a flavoursome chicken or beef stock is not difficult to make, and if onions and garlic are triggers for you, they can be omitted from the recipe.

	uncooked beef or chicken bones (brown beef bones first for richer flavour)	
4	celery stalks, chopped	4
2	medium carrots, chopped	2
2	medium onions, chopped	2
½ tsp	each oregano and thyme	½ tsp
2 tsp	chopped fresh parsley	2 tsp
2	bay leaves	2
2	cloves garlic	2
1 tbsp	salt	1 tbsp
8	peppercorns	8
4	whole cloves	4

Put the bones in a large deep saucepan over medium-high heat. Add all the remaining ingredients and cover with cold water. (If omitting onions and garlic, add an extra bay leaf and another carrot or parsnip). Bring to boil, reduce the heat and simmer, covered, for 4-6 hours. Strain into a large bowl. Discard the bones and vegetables. Leave to cool, then cover and chill overnight. Remove any surface fat before using.
Makes about 4 litres/6 pints.

Kitchen Pointer: This stock can be stored in batches in the freezer and used as the base for many homemade soups.

NUTRIENTS

Contains less than 10 calories per 250 ml/9 fl oz and trace amounts of protein, fat and carbohydrates.

Fish Stock

This versatile stock can be kept in the fridge for up to five days or frozen for up to six months.

3 litres	water	5 pints
250 ml	dry white wine	9 fl oz
2 kg	fish trimmings, washed	4 lb
2	celery stalks, sliced	2
1	onion, sliced	1
2 tbsp	lemon juice	2 tbsp
6	peppercorns	6
4	fresh parsley sprigs	4
2	fresh thyme sprigs or ½ tsp dried	2

Bring the water and wine to boil in a large deep saucepan over high heat. Add the fish trimmings, celery and onion.

Add all the remaining ingredients. When the water returns to the boil, reduce the heat so that the stock is barely simmering. Simmer for 2½-3 hours.

Strain the stock, extracting as much liquid as possible from solids. Discard solids and leave to cool before chilling or freezing.

Makes 3 litres/5 pints.

This recipe is FREE of the following triggers (marked ✔)

Caffeine ✔
Chocolate ✔
Citrus fruits
Red wine ✔
Aged cheese ✔
MSG & Nitrates ✔
Aspartame ✔
Nuts ✔
Onions & Garlic
Yeast ✔

NUTRIENTS

Contains less than 10 calories per 250 ml/9 fl oz and trace amounts of protein, fat and carbohydrates.

Hollandaise Sauce

Serve this sauce over poached salmon (see p. 57), Eggs Benedict or asparagus.

(see p. 57)

6	egg yolks	6
2 tbsp	lemon juice	2 tbsp
225 g	butter, melted	8 oz
4 tbsp	hot water	4 tbsp
pinch	cayenne pepper	pinch
	salt	

Put the egg yolks in the top part of a double boiler or in a bowl placed over a saucepan of hot, but not boiling, water. Beat the egg yolks with a wire whisk until smooth.

Add the lemon juice and gradually whisk in the melted butter, adding it in a thin stream.

Slowly stir in hot water, cayenne pepper and salt to taste. Keep stirring for about 1 minute or until the sauce has thickened.

Serve immediately.

Makes about 500 ml/18 fl oz.

This recipe is FREE of the following triggers (marked ✔)

Caffeine ✔
Chocolate ✔
Citrus fruits
Red wine ✔
Aged cheese ✔
MSG & Nitrates ✔
Aspartame ✔
Nuts ✔
Onions & Garlic ✔
Yeast ✔

PER SERVING
(2 TABLESPOON SERVING)

Kcals	103
g fat	11
g protein	1
g carbohydrate	trace

Homemade Soy Sauce

Most commercially made soy sauce contains MSG, a common trigger for migraine. If you cannot find naturally brewed soy sauce, you might want to consider this recipe. This sauce can be used as a substitute for soy sauce.

175 g	beef drippings from a roast	6 oz
4 tbsp	water	4 tbsp
	sea salt	

Next time you roast a piece of beef, instead of making gravy, save the drippings. After the drippings are cool, skim off the fat.

Mix the beef drippings with the water, and add sea salt to taste.

Store this sauce in an airtight container in the freezer, for up to three months.

This recipe is FREE of the following triggers (marked ✔)

Caffeine ✓
Chocolate ✓
Citrus fruits ✓
Red wine ✓
Aged cheese ✓
MSG & Nitrates ✓
Aspartame ✓
Nuts ✓
Onions & Garlic ✓
Yeast ✓

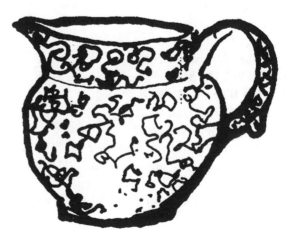

NUTRIENTS

1 tablespoon contains less than 10 Kcals and very small amounts of protein and carbohydrates.

Resources Directory

USEFUL ORGANIZATIONS

Migraine Action Association
178a High Road
Byfleet
Surrey KT14 7ED
Helpline 01932 352 468
Admin 01932 352 468
www.migraine.org.uk
The Migraine Action Association (formerly the British Migraine Association) is a registered charity with over 17,000 members and aims to bridge the gap between the migraine sufferer and the medical world by providing information on all aspects of the condition and its management. The Association is committed to raising general awareness of the condition and provides information; leaflets and newsletters are distributed to clinics, hospitals, libraries and doctors' surgeries throughout the country.
The Association has 3 main aims:
- To provide information and positive reassurance, understanding and encouragement to migraine sufferers and their families
- To encourage and support research and investigation into migraine, its causes, diagnosis, prevention and treatment
- To gather and pass on information about treatments available for the control and relief of migraine and to facilitate an exchange of information on the subject
Offers a telephone helpline, a quarterly newsletter and numerous leaflets on all aspects of migraine. Members participate in research and product trials.

Migraine Trust
45 Great Ormond Street
London WC1N 3HZ
Helpline 020 7831 4818
Admin 020 7831 4818
www.migrainetrust.org
A UK Charity with over 40,000 members which provides good information and services for people with migraine and their doctors. Runs a telephone helpline for sufferers Mon-Fri, 9-5pm. Has local groups support network. The Migraine Trust has a growing network of branches throughout the UK. All branches are run by volunteers with direct experience of migraine. Branches offer:
- Support
- Information and advice
- Visiting speakers

- Publicity work raising the profile of migraine
- Mini-conferences
- Fund-raising events

British Association for the Study of Headache
www.bash.org.uk
BASH has the mission statement 'To relieve those affected by the burdens of headache'. It is an important research organisation in the UK. The site tells you what BASH is doing, about the conferences it organises, and how to get in touch.

OUCH U.K.
The Organisation for the Understanding of Cluster Headache. www.ouch-uk.org

JAMA Migraine Information Centre
www.ama-assn.org/special/migraine
This is a special site of the Journal of the American Medical Association home page that has up to date information on migraine. It also has conference reports and background briefings, as well as the latest literature and a list of websites on migraine that JAMA staff found useful.

International Headache Society
www.i-h-s.org
An important international society for migraine. The site lets you become a member.

World Headache Alliance
www.w-h-a.org
This is an international association of patient groups which represent and provide support for headache sufferers. Useful for those who have migraines, and professionals.

The Migraine Association of Canada
www.migraine.ca

Other useful links from the USA

Migraine Disability Assessment Scale (MIDAS)
www.midas-migraine.net
This site allows the MIDAS scale to be downloaded for use on your computer.

American Council for Headache Education (ACHE)
www.achenet.org

Migraine Awareness Group: A National Understanding for Migraineurs (MAGNUM)
www.migraines.org

American Academy of Neurology (treatment guidelines)
www.aan.com

National Headache Foundation
www.headaches.org

American Headache Society
www.ahsnet.org

MIGRAINE CLINICS
Patients must first obtain a letter from their GP before asking for an appointment at any of these hospitals or clinics.

Specialist Migraine Centres:

The City of London Migraine Clinic
22 Charterhouse Square, London EC1M 6DX
www.colmc.org.uk
Will also treat their registered patients without an appointment during a migraine attack. This registered medical charity accepts GP referrals from all over the United Kingdom at no charge to the referring doctor. Patients are requested to make a donation.

Princess Margaret Migraine Clinic
Charing Cross Hospital, Fulham Palace Road, London W6 8RF

The National Hospital
Queen Square, London WC1N 3ZG
This is a national referral centre for migraine and all headache problems.

Great Ormond Street Hospital
Great Ormond Street, London WC1
This is a special migraine clinic for children.

Hospital Migraine and Neurology Clinics
Banbury: Dept of Neurology, Horton Hospital, Oxford Road, Banbury, Oxon OX16 9BL
Belfast: Royal Victoria Hospital, Grosvenor Road, Belfast BT12 6BA
Birmingham: The Queen Elizabeth Neurosciences Centre, Edgbaston, Birmingham B15 2TT
Cardiff: University Hospital of Wales, Heath Park, Cardiff CF4 4XW
Dublin: Neurology Department, Beaumont Hospital, Beaumont, Dublin 9

Edinburgh: Western General Hospital, Edinburgh EH4 2XU
Exeter: Royal Devon and Exeter Hospital, Barrack Road, Exeter EX2 5DW
Guildford: Royal Surrey County Hospital, Egerton Road, Guildford, Surrey GU2 5XX
Hull: Hull Royal Infirmary, Nanlaby Road, Hull HU3 2JZ
Ipswich: Department of Clinical Neurology, Ipswich Hospital, Heath Road, Ipswich
    IP4 5PD
Leicester: Department of Neurology, Royal Infirmary, Leicester LE1 5WW

London:
King's College Hospital, Denmark Hill, London SE5
Hammersmith Hospital, Du Cane Road, London W12 0HS
The Royal London Hospital, Whitechapel, London E1 1BB

Manchester: Manchester Royal Infirmary, Oxford Road, Manchester M13 9WL
Oxford: The Radcliffe Infirmary, Woodstock Road, Oxford OX2 6HE
Preston: Royal Preston Hospital, Sharoe Green, Preston PR2 4HT
Sheffield: Royal Hallamshire Hospital, Glossop Road, Sheffield S10 2JF
Sunderland: Sunderland Royal Hospital, Kayll Road, Sunderland SR4 7TP
Wakefield: Pinderfields General Hospital, Aberford Road, Wakefield WF1 4DG
York: York District Hospital, Wigginton Road, York YO3 7HE

Neurology Clinics with an interest in headache
All patients with headache can be referred to neurology outpatient departments of the
local hospitals. The following hospitals have doctors with a special interest in headaches.
Basildon: Basildon, Nether Mayne, Basildon SS16 5NL
Cambridge: Addenbrooke's Hospital, Hill Road, Cambridge CB2 2QQ
Colchester: Neurocare Unit, Colchester General Hospital, Colchester CO4 5JL
Leeds: St. James' University Hospital, Beckett Street, Leeds LS9 7TF
Newcastle-on-Tyne: Royal Victoria Infirmary, Queen Victoria Road, Newcastle-upon-Tyne
    NE1 4LP
Northampton: Northampton General Hospital, Cliftonville, Northampton NN1 5BD
Nottingham: University Hospital, Queen's Medical Centre, Nottingham NG7 2UH
Portsmouth: St Mary's Hospital, Milton Road, Portsmouth PO3 8LD
Romford: Essex Neurosciences Unit, Oldchurch Hospital, Romford RM7 0BE
Southampton: Wessex Neurological Centre, Southampton General Hospital, Tremona
    Road, Southampton SO16 6YD
Stafford: District General and Cannock Chase Hospitals, Weston Road, Stafford ST16 3SA

Paediatric Clinics
Aberdeen: Royal Aberdeen Children's Hospital, Cornhill Road, Aberdeen AB9 2ZG
Hartlepool : Paediatric Department, General Hospital, Holdforth Road, Hartlepool
    TS24 9AX
Stirling: Paediatric Department, Stirling Royal Infirmary, Livilands, Stirling FK8 2AU

Bibliography

Bickerstaff, E.R. *Neurological complications of oral contraceptives.* Oxford: Clarendon Press, 1975.

Bousser M.G., and H. Massiou. "Migraine in the reproductive cycle." In J. Olesen et al, *The Headaches.* New York: Raven Press, 1993.

Critchley, Macdonald. "Migraine: From Cappadocia to Queen Square," in *Background to Migraine* (ed.) Robert Smith. New York: Springer-Verlag, 1967.

Edmeads, John. "History of migraine treatment." Can. *J Clin Pharmacol* 1999; 6 (suppl A), Autumn: 5A–8A.

Edmeads J., H. Findlay, P. Tugwell et al. "Impact of migraine and tension-type headache on life-style, consulting behaviour, and medication use: a Canadian population survey." *Can. J Neurol Sci* 1993; 20:131–137.

Epstein, M.T., J.M. Hockaday, and T.D. Hockaday. "Migraine and reproductive hormones throughout the menstrual cycle." *The Lancet* 1975; 1(7906):543–548.

Ferrari, M.D. The Economic Burden of Migraine to Society. *Pharmacoeconomics* 1998; 13:667–676.

Gilmour, H. and K. Wilkins. *Statistics Canada, Health Reports 2001*; Vol. 12, No. 2. Catalogue 82-003.

Goadsby, Peter et al. *Headache in Clinical Practice,* Oxford: Isis Medical Media Ltd., 1998.

Hu, X.H., et al. "Burden of Migraine in the United States: Disability and Economic Costs." *Archives of International Medicine* 1999; 159: 813-818.

Kudrow, L. "The relationship of headache frequency to hormone use in migraine." *Headache* 1975; 15 (Apr):36–40.

Lipton R.B., and W.F. Stewart. "Migraine in the United States: Epidemiology and Health Care Use." *Neurology* 1993; 43 (suppl 3):6–10.

McKim, A. Elizabeth. "Ancient Migraine." *Headlines* 8-3, 1999: 1–5.

O'Brien, B., R. Goeree, and D. Streiner. "Prevalence of Migraine Headache in Canada: A Population-Based Survey." *Int J Epidemiol* 1994; 23:1020–1026.

Osterhaus J.T., R.J. Townsend, B. Gandek et al. "Measuring the functional status and well-being of patients with migraine headache." *Headache* 1994; 34:337–343.

Pryse-Phillips W., H. Findlay, P. Tugwell, et al. "A Canadian Population Survey on the Clinical, Epidemiologic and Societal Impact of Migraine and Tension-Type Headache." *Can J Neurol Sci* 1992; 19:333–339.

Silberstein S.D. "Migraine and women: The link between headache and hormones." *Postgraduate Medicine* 1995; 97(4):147–153.

Silberstein S.D., and R.B. Lipton. "Headache epidemiology: Emphasis on migraine." *Neurology Clinics* 1996; 14:421–434.

Simon, Maurice (ed.) *The Babylonian Talmud: Seder Nashim* Vol. 3. London: Soncino, 1936.

South, Valerie. *Migraine.* Toronto: Key Porter Books, 1994.

Stewart W.F., R.B. Lipton, et al. "Prevalence of migraine headache in the United States: Relation to age, income, race and other socio-demographic factors." *Jama* 1992; 267(1):64–69.

Index

A

acetaminophen, xii, xvi
acetylsalicylic acid (ASA),
  xii, xvi
acupuncture, xviii
additives, xvi
alcohol (trigger), xxi
Allspice Roasted Bananas,
  93
Almond Crescents, 111
amines, xx, xxi
analgesics, x
appetisers and snacks
  Grilled Gravadlax with
    Mustard Dill Sauce, 9
  Herbed Pitta Crisps, 3
  Houmous, 5
  Oatcakes, 2
  Prawn Pastries, 7
  Shiitake Perogies with
    Sweet Ginger Sauce, 6
  Vegetable Platter with
    Olive Oil Dip, 4
Apple Cobbler, 90
Apple Pancakes, 89
artificial sweeteners, xxii
Asparagus Spears with
  Apple, Egg and Poppy
  Seed Dressing, 72
Aspartame, xvi
atypical migraine, ix
aura, viii, ix, xiii

B

Baked Halibut with Dill
  Crust and Red Pepper
  Sauce, 62
basilar (artery) migraine, ix
beef
  Swedish Meatballs, 47
beef stock, 122
beta-blockers, xvii
beverages
  Fruit Punch, 117
  Hot Spiced Punch, 118
  Migraine Mellower, 116
  Mint Julep, 114

Mulled Cider, 119
Peppermint Cooler, 115
Bickerstaff's migraine, ix
biofeedback, xviii
Black-Eyed Bean Salad with
  Peppers, 24
Blueberry Maple Pie with
  Warmed Maple Syrup, 94
breads
  Buttermilk Scones, 85
  Corn Bread, 86
  Courgette Bread, 87
  Healthy Scones, 83
  Irish Scones, 84
  Never-Fail Scones, 82
breakfast, xxiii
bulgur
  Bulgar and Green Bean
    Salad with Herbed
    Vinaigrette, 78
Buttermilk Scones, 85

C

caffeine (trigger), xv, xx
cakes and pies
  Blueberry Maple Pie with
    Warmed Maple Syrup,
    94
  Cranberry Carrot Cake with
    Cream Cheese Frosting,
    100
  Ginger Pound Cake, 98
  Maple Syrup Cake, 99
  Old-Fashioned
    Butterscotch Pie, 97
  Peach Sponge, 96
calcitonin gene-related
  peptide (CGRP), ix
calcium channel blockers,
  xvii
Carob Chip Cookies, 109
Charred Courgettes with
  Herbs, Garlic and Ricotta,
  73
cheeses (trigger), xxi
Chicken Kebabs with
  Homemade Barbecue

Sauce, 41
chicken stock, 122
children, migraine in, xi
Chinese Noodle Salad with
  Roasted Aubergine, 30
chiropractic, xviii
chocolate (trigger), xvi, xxi
cigarette smoke, xvi
classic migraine. See
  migraine with aura
citrus fruits (trigger), xvi, xxi
cluster headaches, x, xiii
cognitive-behavioural
  therapy (CBT), xviii
common migraine. See
  migraine without aura
complementary therapies,
  xvii
cookies and squares
  Almond Crescents, 111
  Carob Chip Cookies, 109
  Ginger Snaps, 112
  No-Bake Carob-Oatmeal
    Macaroons, 110
  Shortbread, 106
Corn Bread, 86
Courgette Bread, 87
Cranberry Carrot Cake with
  Cream Cheese Frosting, 100
Cream of Mushroom Soup,
  11
Cream of Spinach Soup, 12
Crème Brûlée with
  Rosemary, 102
Curried Chicken with
  Peaches and Coconut, 38
Curried Chicken and Rice
  Salad with Almonds, 25
Curried Winter Vegetable
  Soup, 15

D

daily routine, changes to
  (trigger), xii, xv
dairy products (trigger), xvi,
  xxi
desserts

Allspice Roasted Bananas, 93
Apple Cobbler, 90
Crème Brûlée with Rosemary, 102
Lemon Curd with Shortbread and Raspberry Coulis, 105
Mocha Mousse with Cinnamon Whipped Cream, 107
Moltoff with Fresh Berry Compote, 103
Poached Fruit in Light Syrup with Vanilla Ice Cream and Roasted Almonds, 92
Roasted Pears with Minted Custard, 91
diary (triggers), xxiii
doughnuts
Doughnuts, Wholewheat 108
E
Easy Fish Chowder, 16
environmental triggers, xv
F
familial hemiplegic migraine, ix
feverfew, xviii
Filo-Wrapped Chicken with Mushrooms and Spinach in Citron Vodka Sauce, 45
fish and seafood
Baked Halibut with Dill Crust and Red Pepper Sauce, 62
Easy Fish Chowder, 16
Fresh Tuna with Maple Mustard and Coriander Oil, 53
Grilled Gravadlax with Mustard Dill Sauce, 9
Grilled Salmon Steaks with Mango Strawberry Coriander Chutney, 58
Grilled Prawns with Two Marinades, 65

Herb-Crusted Salmon Fillets, 56
Kedgeree, 55
Lemon Sole with Oranges and Honey, 63
Pan-Fried Trout with Cucumber and Prawn Salsa, 61
Poached Salmon in Rosé, 57
Portuguese Seafood Risotto, 67
Prawn and Carrot Risotto, 66
Prawn Pastries, 7
Salmon Wrapped in Rice Paper in a Yellow Pepper Sauce, 59
Scallops with White Wine and Tarragon Sauce, 64
fish stock, 123
food allergies, xx
food colourings/dyes, xxiii
food trigger diary, xxiii
food triggers, xiv, xix
Fresh Berry Compote, 104
Fresh Tuna with Maple Mustard and Coriander Oil, 53
Fruit Punch, 117
fruits (triggers), xxi
G
Ginger Snaps, 112
Ginger Pound Cake, 98
Grated Root Vegetable Salad with Roasted Apple Dressing, 18
Grilled Gravadlax with Mustard Dill Sauce, 9
Grilled Polenta with Tomato Sauce, 79
Grilled Portobello Mushrooms with Asparagus and Herbed Polenta, 33
Grilled Portobello Mushrooms with Goats' Cheese and Rocket, 23
Grilled Prawns with Two

Marinades, 65
Grilled Salmon Steaks with Mango Strawberry Coriander Chutney, 58
H
headache syndromes, x
Healthy Scones, 83
Herb and Cherry Tabbouleh, 77
Herb-Crusted Salmon Fillets, 56
Herbed Pitta Crisps, 3
Hollandaise Sauce, 124
Homemade Soy Sauce, 125
Homestyle Quick Chicken Curry, 36
Honey-Roasted Lamb Fillet with Green Asparagus and Plantain Mash, 51
hormonal cycles/changes (trigger), xi, xv
hormone replacement therapy (HRT), xv
Hot Spiced Punch, 118
Houmous, 5
hypnotherapy, xviii
I
Irish Scones, 84
J
Japanese-Glazed Chicken, 39
K
Kedgeree, 55
L
Lamb
Honey-Roasted Lamb Fillet with Green Asparagus and Plantain Mash, 51
Quick Lamb Patties, 50
Lasagne (vegetarian), 32
Lemon Curd with Shortbread and Raspberry Coulis, 105
Lemon Sole with Oranges and Honey, 63
M
magnesium, xviii
Maple Syrup Cake, 99
massage, xviii

meatless main courses
Chinese Noodle Salad with Roasted Aubergine, 30
Grilled Portobello Mushrooms with Asparagus and Herbed Polenta, 33
Pasta Salad with Red Peppers and Artichokes, 29
Roasted Wild Mushroom Veggie Burgers, 28
Stir-Fried Fresh Vegetables and Tofu, 34
Vegetable and Cheese Lasagne, 32
medication, x, xi, xiii-xiv, xix
medication-induced headaches, x
menopause, xi, xv
menstrual cycle, xi, xv
menstrually-related migraine, xi
Middle Eastern Salad, 19
migraine
avoiding, checklist, xxiv
causes of, viii
in children, xi
diagnosing, xiii
managing, xvi
non-drug strategies, xvii
resources, 126-129
symptoms, viii, x, xi, xii
triggers, xiv, xix
in women, x
Migraine Mellower, 116
migraine-specific medications, xii
migraine with aura, ix
migraine without aura, ix
Mint Julep, 114
Mocha Mousse with Cinnamon Whipped Cream, 107
Moltoff with Fresh Berry Compote, 103
monosodium glutamate (MSG), xxii

Mulled Cider, 119
Mushrooms and Rice, 75
N
Never-Fail Scones, 82
No-Bake Carob-Oatmeal Macaroons, 110
non-steroidal anti-inflammatory agents (NSAIDs), xi
nuts and seeds (trigger), xxii
O
Oatcakes, 2
oestrogen, xi
Old-Fashioned Butterscotch Pie, 97
Onion Confit, 22
ophthalmoplegic migraine, x
oral contraceptives, xi
P
pancakes
Apple Pancakes, 89
Pancakes, 88
Pan-Fried Trout with Cucumber and Prawn Salsa, 61
pasta
Pasta with Chicken, Asparagus, and Sweet Red Pepper, 40
Pasta Salad with Red Peppers and Artichokes, 29
Vegetable and Cheese Lasagne, 32
Peach Sponge, 96
Peppermint Cooler, 115
Perogies, 6
pies. See cakes and pies
Poached Chicken with Wild Rice and Baby Vegetables, 43
Poached Fruit in Light Syrup with Vanilla Ice Cream and Roasted Almonds, 92
Poached Salmon in Rosé Wine, 57
polenta
Grilled Polenta with

Tomato Sauce, 79
Grilled Portobello Mushrooms with Asparagus and Herbed Polenta, 33
pork
Pork Fillet with Fresh Tomato Sauce, 49
Sweet and Sour Pork Chops, 48
Portuguese Seafood Risotto, 67
poultry
Chicken Kebabs with Homemade Barbecue Sauce, 41
Curried Chicken with Peaches and Coconut, 38
Curried Chicken and Rice Salad with Almonds, 25
Filo-Wrapped Chicken with Mushrooms and Spinachin Citron Vodka Sauce, 45
Homestyle Quick Chicken Curry, 36
Japanese-Glazed Chicken, 39
Pasta with Chicken, Asparagus, and Sweet Red Pepper, 40
Poached Chicken with Wild Rice and Baby Vegetables, 43
Roast Duck with Spiced Honey, 44
Simple Chicken Kiev, 37
Prawn and Carrot Risotto, 66
Prawn Pastries, 7
preventive medications, xvii
progesterone, xi
Pumpkin Bisque, 13
Q
Quick Lamb Patties, 50
R
Raspberry Coulis, 105
rebound headaches, x
relaxation therapy, xvii

riboflavin, xviii
rice
  Curried Chicken and Rice
    Salad with Almonds, 25
  Mushrooms and Rice, 75
  Portuguese Seafood
    Risotto, 67
  Prawn and Carrot Risotto,
    66
  Steamed Basmati Rice with
    Crisp Potatoes, Sumac
    and Cumin, 76
Roast Duck with Spiced
  Honey, 44
Roasted New Potatoes
  with Herbs, 74
Roasted Pears with Minted
  Custard, 91
Roasted Potato Salad, 17
Roasted Vegetable Medley,
  71
Roasted Wild Mushroom
  Veggie Burgers, 28
S
salads
  Black-Eyed Bean Salad
    with Peppers, 24
  Bulgur and Green Bean
    Salad with Herbed
    Vinaigrette, 78
  Chinese Noodle Salad with
    Roasted Aubergine, 30
  Curried Chicken and Rice
    Salad with Almonds, 25
  Grated Root Vegetable
    Salad with Roasted Apple
    Dressing, 18
  Grilled Portobello
    Mushrooms with Goats'
    Cheese and Rocket, 23
  Middle Eastern Salad, 19
  Pasta Salad with Red
    Peppers and Artichokes,
    29
  Roasted Potato Salad, 17
  Toasted Creamy Goats'
    Cheese with Onion
    Confit, 22

Warm Spinach Salad with
  Prawns, 26
Warmed Goats' Cheese
  Salad with Grilled
  Vegetables, 20
Salmon Wrapped in Rice
  Paper in a Yellow Pepper
  Sauce, 59
sauces
  Hollandaise Sauce, 124
  Homemade Soy Sauce,
    125
  Mustard Dill Sauce, 9
Scallops with White Wine
  and Tarragon Sauce, 64
scones, 82, 83, 84, 85
seafood. See fish and
  seafood
serotonin, xvii
Shiitake Perogies with Sweet
  Ginger Sauce, 6
Shortbread, 106
Simple Chicken Kiev, 37
sleep, changes in (trigger), xv
snacks. See appetisers and
  snacks
soups (See also stocks)
  Cream of Mushroom Soup,
    11
  Cream of Spinach Soup, 12
  Curried Winter Vegetable
    Soup, 15
  Easy Fish Chowder, 16
  Pumpkin Bisque, 13
  Vichyssoise, 14
soy sauce (homemade),
  125
Steamed Basmati Rice with
  Crisp Potatoes, Sumac and
  Cumin, 76
Stir-Fried Fresh Vegetables
  and Tofu, 34
Stir-Fried Peppers and Bean
  Sprouts, 70
stocks
  Chicken or Beef Stock, 122
  Fish Stock, 123
  Vegetable Stock, 121

Sweet and Sour Pork Chops,
  48
Swedish Meatballs, 47
syncopal migraine, ix
T
Tabbouleh, 77
tension headache, viii
Toasted Creamy Goats'
  with Onion Confit, 22
triggers, xvi, xix
V
Vegetable and Cheese
  Lasagne, 32
Vegetable Platter with Olive
  Oil Dip (Pinzimonio), 4
vegetable side dishes
  Asparagus Spears with
    Apple, Egg and Poppy
    Seed Dressing, 72
  Charred Courgettes with
    Herbs, Garlic and
    Ricotta, 73
  Herb and Cherry
    Tabbouleh, 77
  Mushrooms and Rice, 75
  Roasted New Potatoes with
    Herbs, 74
  Roasted Vegetable Medley,
    71
  Steamed Basmati Rice with
    Crisp Potatoes, Sumac
    and Cumin, 76
  Stir-Fried Peppers and
    Bean Sprouts, 70
vegetable stock, 121
Vichychoisse, 14
W
Warm Spinach Salad with
  Prawns, 26
Warmed Goats' Cheese
  Salad with Grilled
  Vegetables, 20
Wholewheat Doughnuts,
  108
women, migraine in, x